Measuring Outcomes:
Data Analysis Made Easy

Deborah K. Wall RN, BSN, MA

Precept Press, Chicago
Division of Bonus Books, Inc.

Wall, Deborah K.
    Measuring outcomes: data analysis made easy/Deborah K. Wall.
        p. cm.
    Includes bibliographical references and index.
    ISBN 0-944496-52-0
    1. Outcome assessment (Medical care)—Methodology. I. Title.
    [DNLM: 1. Outcome and Process Assessment (Health Care)
    2. Research Design. 3. Data Collection. 4. Statistics—methods.
    5. Cost-Benefit Analysis—methods. W 84.3 W187m 1997]
    R853.087W35 1997
    362.1 ' 0285—dc21
    DNLM/DCL
    for Library of Congress   97-17398
                                                                          CIP

Precept Press
Division of Bonus Books. Inc.
160 East Illinois Street
Chicago, Illinois 60611

Table of Contents

1

Planning for Data Analysis

In recent years, the health care industry has obtained a new appreciation of statistical thinking regarding quality, costs and services. By being able to statistically analyze clinical and administrative processes, many improvements can be identified and results can be quantified.

This program covers statistical thinking and techniques for performance improvement professionals, clinicians and administrators. **Statistical thinking makes people better managers, analysts, health care providers, administrators and so on.** It is a formal framework for systematic clarification of ambiguous and uncertain processes and provides efficiencies of thought. The end result is improved design of patient care processes and cost savings. Statistics, despite its reputation as an abstract and difficult subject, is an eminently practical one. To put analysis in proper context, both study design and data collection issues will be addressed.

Study Design

Before any data can be collected and analyzed, a study needs to be designed. One of the major objectives of data analysis is to prove something. This objective gives a clearly defined purpose for collecting data. To design a clinical study:

1. State the reason for the study of a topic

2. Define the problem being investigated

3. Select a population to include in the study

4. Choose a methodology for the study

5. Calculate sample size requirements

6. Determine data analysis methods

7. Formulate conclusions

Each of these will be discussed in the following sections.

Reasons for Collecting Data

Before initiating a clinical, quality or resource study, the reason for collecting data needs to be understood. Otherwise, you might collect data that does not meet the main purpose of the study in the first place.

There are three main reasons for collecting data. **The first is to predict future behavior of people or processes.** For example, data about the initiation of antibiotics prior to surgery and the incidence of surgical wound infections can be used to predict a patient's chance of developing an infection if antibiotics are not administered. Studies which are designed to predict future behaviors frequently use inferential statistics to make predictions based on the probability of a certain behavior or outcome occurring.

The second reason for collecting data is to **detect changes in a process.** For example, at a local hospital the average length of stay for patients with community-acquired bacterial pneumonia is 5.2 days. However, during the month of December, the average length of stay reduced to 4.5 days. This shift downward relative to the previously observed behavior might trigger investigation into the reasons for the reduction.

The final reason for data collection is **to share or communicate information.** For example, if a sequence plot graph showing the number of medication errors which occur every day is posted in the pharmacy and updated every day, pharmacists can see the effects of the medication distribution process.

Reasons for Collecting Data

- ◆ **Predict future behaviors**

- ◆ **Detect change in a process**

- ◆ **Share or communicate information**

Problem Definition

Problem definition is simply a statement of the purpose for the study. This problem is usually stated as a question or as a desired patient outcome. For example, the reason to study the care of patients with congestive heart failure is to reduce the length of stay, or reduce the incidence of pulmonary edema, or reduce the number of readmissions during a specific timeframe. These reasons are converted to study questions which ask how can the length of stay be reduced, or how can the incidence of pulmonary edema be reduced. Without this purpose, data collection is just a meaningless activity. A clearly defined purpose provides the context for data analysis.

Once a problem has been identified, hypotheses about how the problem may be solved need to be developed. A hypothesis states a belief (educated guess) about the relationship between specific data elements. Forming hypotheses is important because they provide the logic for consensus building, direct information requirements and guide the selection of analytical tools.

Hypotheses state the relationship between clinical process interventions and the desired patient outcomes. For example, clinicians state a hypothesis regarding the relationship between the timing of an antibiotic and the length of stay for patients with a principal diagnosis of pneumonia.

Hypotheses State Relationships
Being Tested During Clinical Study

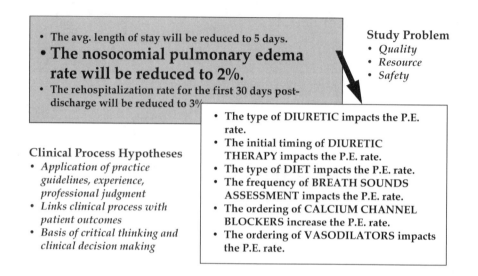

- The avg. length of stay will be reduced to 5 days.
- **The nosocomial pulmonary edema rate will be reduced to 2%.**
- The rehospitalization rate for the first 30 days post-discharge will be reduced to 3%

Study Problem
- *Quality*
- *Resource*
- *Safety*

Clinical Process Hypotheses
- *Application of practice guidelines, experience, professional judgment*
- *Links clinical process with patient outcomes*
- *Basis of critical thinking and clinical decision making*

- The type of DIURETIC impacts the P.E. rate.
- The initial timing of DIURETIC THERAPY impacts the P.E. rate.
- The type of DIET impacts the P.E. rate.
- The frequency of BREATH SOUNDS ASSESSMENT impacts the P.E. rate.
- The ordering of CALCIUM CHANNEL BLOCKERS increase the P.E. rate.
- The ordering of VASODILATORS impacts the P.E. rate.

Once the problem definition is complete and hypotheses are stated, it is time to define the study's population.

Select Population

Population definition and selection is an important part of study design because it facilitates consistent decisions by data collectors regarding whom to include in a study, identifies the sample sizes needed and describes to whom the conclusions can be applied. The objective is to create a homogeneous sample, enhancing the accuracy and validity of analysis. An example of a population description for a fractured hip study might be:

> All patients over the age of 65 years admitted through the emergency department with a primary diagnosis of closed intertrochanteric or subtrochanteric fracture (ICD-9-CM: 820.21, 820.22) due to trauma. All patients will receive surgical intervention for fractures. Patients with active infectious processes or malignancies will be excluded from the study.

Study Methodology

The study methodology consists of at least two parts. One is the type of study being conducted and the other is defining the type of data elements in a study.

Types of Studies

The simplest way of collecting data is to record outcomes generated by the process as it evolves. These outcomes can be measured systematically at predetermined instants. This entire process is called **simple observation**. Many occurrence screening and utilization review programs use a simple observation method of evaluating the effectiveness and efficiency of a clinical process.

A second type of study is the **sample survey**. In reality, collecting data can be time consuming and expensive. To facilitate maximum information at minimum cost, most health care organizations use a **sample survey** study design. The sample survey consists of selecting a sample of elements for measurement from a universe of elements. *A universe refers to the collection of all elements of interest*, such as patients who have congestive heart failure during a specified time period. A sample is a collection of elements drawn from the universe and studied by collecting data, such as answers to questions, observation of certain behaviors and so forth. For example, to determine if a medical record meets the pertinence of medical records requirements, a questionnaire is developed asking specific questions about the timing of completion and the content of a patient's chart.

Study Methodology: Sample Survey

- **Selecting a sample of elements for measurement from a universe of elements**

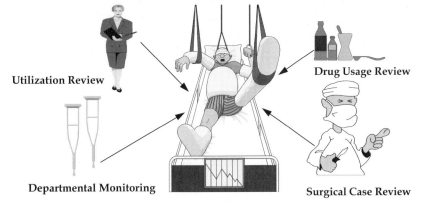

Utilization Review

Drug Usage Review

Departmental Monitoring

Surgical Case Review

Another type of study is an **experiment**, which is the study of the effects of change in a limited environment that is, to some degree, under the control of the experimenter. Although experiments help explain the effects of changes, their results cannot always be immediately generalized to practical situations because the control exercised in the experiment may not be possible in the real world. However, field experiments in real-world settings, such as a drug trial with experimental medications, produce results more readily applicable to immediate problems. Using the experimental approach to determine causation in the real world is called **quasi-experimentation**.

For a study to be considered experimental there needs to be at least a treatment, an outcome measure, units of assignment and some comparison from which change can be inferred and hopefully attributed to the treatment. There are three types of quasi-experiments: nonequivalent group designs, interrupted time-series designs and correlational-designs.

Nonequivalent group designs are typically those in which responses of a treatment group and a comparison group are measured before and after a treatment. This would be the case where two groups of patients are compared to each other and outcome data is collected at the beginning and end of the inpatient service. For example, patients with congestive heart failure can be divided into groups which receive ACE inhibitors and those which do not receive this medication. By comparing the severity levels of each group at the time of admission and then at discharge, clinicians are using nonequivalent group design to determine if ACE inhibitors is a causal force of severity level.

Interrupted time-series design is used when clinicians compare measures of performance taken at many time intervals before a treatment with measures taken at many intervals afterwards. For example, the length of stay for patients with congestive heart failure is measured for three months prior to pathway implementation and then for three months after implementation. The comparison between the lengths of stay will help determine if causal inferences can be made for the developed pathway.

Finally, **correlational-designs**, also called passive observational methods, most often refers to efforts at causal inference based on measures taken all at one time, with differential levels of both effects and exposures to presumed causes, being measured as they occur naturally, without any experimental interventions. For example, comparing the length of stay between groups of patients who receive ACE inhibitors and those who do not receive ACE inhibitors.

Although any of the three types of studies, simple observation, sample survey or experiment, can be used to measure quality and to monitor clinical processes, a decision needs to be made regarding what type of study will meet the needs of the organization within the available resources and time constraints.

Types of Data

One thing to remember is that we seldom have complete knowledge of a process, nor can we expect to exercise complete control over every step in a process. Fortunately, most processes can be managed by exercising control at just a few critical steps. **A key ingredient in managing and improving health care processes is to stay in touch with the critical steps by collecting relevant measurements.** Such measurements are called **data**.

Data should be collected systematically over a long period of time from the truly critical steps of a process. **Studies of the evolution of a process over time are called longitudinal studies.** More precisely, a longitudinal study consists of:

- Collection of data from a process over time
- Comparison of data from different time periods
- Documentation of variation over time
- Evaluation of changes in behavior of the process

Measuring critical pathway compliance and variance tracking is an example of a longitudinal study. By thinking longitudinally, we focus on those aspects of the process critical for decision making. By limiting our attention to the points that make the most difference, we work at peak efficiency, avoiding wasted effort.

Process Data

Process data is one of the basic types of data found in the health care industry. **This data relates to the sequence of steps taken by caregivers to cure illness or improve the health of a patient.** To measure the quality of a process, data must be collected. Types of data are measures of the characteristics of a process. For example, to monitor the process of treating pneumonia, the number and timing of chest x-rays are recorded for each patient with a diagnosis of pneumonia. By aggregating the data, clinicians can understand at least one process variable in the treatment of pneumonia.

Since a process is a sequence of steps taken to achieve a goal, the scientific study of a process seeks to model each step and the relationships among the steps. A successful model yields understanding of the fundamental causes of the variations in the process. Activities leading to such an understanding are called process analyses.

Ideally, a model also yields accurate predictions of the future behavior of the process. If so, the model can be used as a basis for process control. Control may mean keeping the process outcomes near a predetermined "target" so the output from the process is dependable. This kind of control, which is also called process regulation, is typical in laboratory calibration and process improvement efforts.

Continuous Data

To be analyzed statistically, data must be numerical or coded numerically. Even things that are not strictly measurable must be reduced to cold figures. For example, patient satisfaction is captured using an numeric rating system instead of a series of statements. Numeric measurements give us a concrete handle on problems that no amount of speculation can replace.

Continuous data is generally classified using an ordinal scale because some observations have more or are greater than other observations. For example, the dyspnea level of a patient with congestive heart failure is recorded using an ordinal scale from one to four. If the continuous data describes the quantity of something, then a numerical scale is used to describe the type of data being collected. For example, the temperature of a patient, twenty four hours after surgery is a quantitative observation and can be recorded on a numerical scale.

Categorical Data

Another important type of data is categorical data, data that is arranged in classes or categories. These categories are determined by classifying elements into groups according to a common attribution. For example, all people who have congestive heart failure and receive ACE inhibitors are in the same category. By counting the number of elements or cases in this category we are dealing with categorical data.

Nominal scales are frequently used to present categorical data or qualitative observations. This is because they describe a quality of the element. Nominal data generally are described in terms of percentages or proportions.

When a collection of data values becomes available for analysis, it is important to understand the basic characteristics of the collection. This understanding helps determine the best type of analysis to use on the available data.

Sampling

An important study design issue in causal research is the selection and size of a sample. This issue is important because it impacts the level of confidence in the inferences made from available data and promotes study validity.

Sample size is influenced by the population's degree of homogeneity, the desired level of confidence and/or the type of statistical test being used.

Sampling: A Collection of Elements Drawn from the Universe

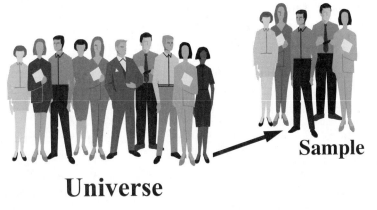

Sample

Universe

Sample size influenced by homogeneity, level of confidence, and type of statistical test

The homogeneity of the population is the degree of sameness within a population. For example, if 90 percent of patients with pneumonia receive a chest x-ray in the emergency department, there is a high degree of homogeneity. However, if 20 different antibiotic regimens are used to treat patients with pneumonia then there is a low degree of homogeneity.

The level of confidence is the probability of an incorrect assumption being accepted. For example, clinicians may want to be 95 percent sure that giving an antibiotic two hours prior to an incision will reduce the probability of the patient developing a surgical wound infection.

The type of statistical test influences the sample size because certain tests have minimum population sizes established. For example, to perform a z-test, which determines if there is a difference between two different populations, a minimum sample size for each population is 30.

Samples must be selected randomly, regardless of their size. Every case must have an equal chance of being included in the sample in order to provide an accurate reflection of the total population and serve as an adequate foundation for statistical tests. Randomization promotes "external" validity. Clinicians can use various methods for choosing cases, including simple random, systematic random, stratified random and cluster sampling.

1. **Simple Random Sample:** A portion of items (cases) selected from a population in a manner, such as using a number table, which ensures all items have an equal chance or probability of being chosen.

2. **Systematic Random Sample:** A sampling method where every nth number of items is selected for the sample. "N" is a predetermined constant number of cases. For example, every seventh case will be included in the sample.

3. **Stratified Random Sample:** Selecting a portion of a population by subdividing it according to specified characteristics, then randomly choosing cases from each sub-group.

4. **Cluster Random Sample:** A two stage sampling process which first subdivides the population into groups or clusters according to a specific characteristic, then a random sample of clusters is chosen. A portion of subjects within each cluster are selected. This sampling method is most often used in epidemiological research and commonly based on geographic areas or districts.

There are many formulas for computing adequate sample size. These formulas are based on the homogeneity of the population, the desired level of confidence and the power of the study. To estimate the approximate sample size for a study comparing the mean in one group to a standard value, four questions must be answered:

- What level of significance related to the null hypothesis is desired? The smaller the level of significance the larger the sample size.

- How high should the chances be of detecting an actual difference? The larger the sample size, the higher the chance of detecting an actual difference.

- How large should the difference be between the means in order for the difference to have clinical importance? The larger the difference between the groups, the smaller the required sample size.

- What is a good estimate of the standard deviation in the population? The more homogenous the populations are the smaller the sample size because the cases will be distributed among fewer groups.

Data Analysis

Once data has been collected, clinicians need to be able to tell a story using the collected data. This story needs to describe the current situation, show how the elements or factors relate to one another and predict what will probably happen in the future. The storytelling method is called data analysis. There are two basic types of data analysis, descriptive and inferential.

Descriptive analysis identifies the common attributes of a given set of data and focuses on central tendencies, variations and frequency measurements. These measurements are important because they allow for summarization of information and provide essential data required for more sophisticated tests.

Inferential analysis allows clinicians to test their established beliefs by making comparisons among different populations and correlating the interventions with outcomes. Inferential statistics help explain why a certain event occurs.

Formulate Conclusions

The final component of a study is the formulation of a conclusion. This conclusion or decision is based on the significance of available evidence and the clinician's confidence about that evidence.

To understand how study conclusions are made, clinicians need to be aware of the use of null hypotheses. A null hypothesis (H_O) is a statement claiming that there is no difference between the hypothesis value and the population. The alternative hypothesis (H_1) is a statement which disagrees with this statement. For example, clinicians may believe that giving an antibiotic less than two hours prior to surgery will reduce the surgical wound infection rate. To test this statement, a null hypothesis is formulated which states "giving an antibiotic less than two hours prior to surgery **does not** reduce the surgical wound infection rate." The alternative hypothesis is then "giving an antibiotic less than two hours prior to surgery reduces the surgical wound infection rate." If the null hypothesis is rejected as a result of sample evidence, then the alternative hypothesis is the conclusion. However, if there is not insufficient evidence to reject the null hypothesis, it is retained but not "accepted." The reason the null hypothesis is not accepted is that scientists argue that a better study may reject the null hypothesis. Therefore, clinicians do not "accept" the null hypothesis from current evidence, but merely state that it cannot be rejected. Statistical hypothesis testing seems to be somewhat reversed from our non-statistical thinking because the focus is on disproving a belief instead of proving a hypothesis.

There are two types of errors which can occur when making a conclusion. The first kind of error is called a **type I error** and relates to rejecting the null hypothesis when it is true. It is also known as an α error. The second kind of error is a **type II error**, and it is an error which occurs when a null hypothesis is not rejected when it is false. A type II error is a β error.

Related to hypothesis testing and type of errors is power. Power is defined as the probability of rejecting the null hypothesis when it is false or of concluding the alternative hypothesis when it is true. This is the capability of a study to detect a given difference of a given size if the difference really exists. Power is calculated as $1-\beta$.

TABLE 1. Correct decisions and errors in hypothesis testing

	True Situation: Difference exists (H$_1$)	True Situation: No difference (H$_0$)
Difference exists (Conclusion: Reject H$_0$)	* (**Power or** $1-\beta$)	I (Type I error, or α error)
No Difference exists (Conclusion: Do not reject H$_0$)	II (Type II error, or β error)	*

2

Descriptive Analysis
Made Easy

Measures of Central Tendencies

To begin data analysis it is important to understand how data is distributed within a selected population or sample size. This distribution will allow clinicians to describe the population in numerical (nominal) terms. Numeric or frequency methods of analysis are often called descriptive statistics. **Descriptive statistics identify the common attributes of a given set of data and focus on central tendencies, variations and frequency measurements.** These measurements are important because they allow for summarization of information and provide essential data required for more sophisticated tests.

Frequency Distribution

When summarizing raw data, it is useful to distribute the data into groups or categories and determine the number of individuals belonging to each group. By counting the number of cases in each category (categorical data) we are determining the frequency distribution. **Frequency distributions show a clear "overall" picture from which vital relationships between data elements can become evident.** Frequency distributions should be used to demonstrate "Patterns of Care."

Examples of patterns of care for Electrolytes are "Pre-admission only," "Day of Surgery" and "Pre-admission and First Post-operative Day." Once patterns of care are identified, analysts need to count the number of cases (or frequency) which demonstrate each pattern of care. The result of these counts is the frequency distribution. It is important to remember that the sum of each category does not exceed the total number of cases in the sample.

To formulate a frequency distribution, clinicians or analysts should:

Step 1.   Select categories for stratifying data

Step 2.   Sum the number of values in each group

EXAMPLE: Using the data in the first case study calculate the frequency distribution for patients who receive a type of vasodilator.

Step 1.   The stratification of this group are (1) patients without a vasodilator (2) patients receiving Nitro (3) patients receiving Isordil and (4) patients Nitro and Isordil.

Step 2.   Calculate the number of values in each group

TABLE 2.

Category of Groups	Frequency Distribution
Patient without vasodilator	12
Patients receiving Nitro	11
Patients receiving Isordil	4
Patients receiving Isordil and Nitro	3

EXERCISE: Using the data in the first case study calculate the frequency distribution for the time the patient receives their first dose of vasodilator.

Step 1.   The stratification of this group are (1) patients without a vasodilator (2) patients receiving the first dose on 0-2 hrs (3) patients receiving the first dose Day one and (4) patients receiving the first dose on Day two.

Step 2.   Calculate the number of values in each group

TABLE 3.

Category of Groups	Frequency Distribution

Histograms

Histograms are graphic tools for displaying distributions of large sets of data. Histograms group the data into a relatively small number of classes and show the frequencies of the classes. In the statistical literature, several somewhat different displays are called histograms. We distinguish among three types: frequency histograms, relative frequency histograms and density histograms.

Frequency histograms, the most basic histograms, are graphic displays of frequency distributions. All they require is grouping the data into classes, counting the number of observations in each class, and making a plot.

EXAMPLE: Using the data in the frequency distribution example above, develop a frequency histogram.

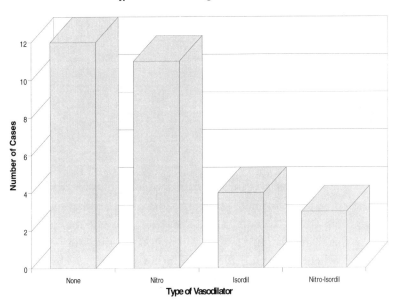

Type of Vasodilator Usage for CHF Patients

EXERCISE: Using the data in the exercise frequency distribution table, plot a frequency histogram.

13			
12			
11			
10			
9			
8			
7			
6			
5			
4			
3			
2			
1			
0			

Dotplots

Another way to display frequency data is called a dotplot, which shows the numerical values along a horizontal scale. If a data value repeats, another dot is placed at the corresponding location along the scale, one dot for each repetition. Statisticians say that a dotplot displays the distribution of the data. **The dotplot is especially useful when displaying the distribution of a relatively small set of numbers.** It shows the position of the data points on a number line and displays frequencies.

Dotplots are useful when displaying the distribution of numeric outcomes for categorical data. For example, displaying the distribution of the length of stays for patients who received different types of vasodilators

EXAMPLE: Using the data in the same data in the case study, plot the length of stay for each data element in each category.

Step 1.   List the length of stay for each case which meets the category criteria in the first column.

Category of Groups	Lengths of Stay Values
Patients without Vasodilators	5, 4, 6, 14, 4, 8, 11, 4, 6, 6, 6, 9
Patients receiving Nitro	7, 5, 7, 9, 5, 4, 3, 8, 5, 5, 4
Patients receiving Isordil	2, 8, 6, 7
Patient receiving Nitro and Isordil	7, 10, 5

Step 2. Write the categories of vasodilators in the left most column.

Step 3. On the bottom row, write the possible lengths of stay from 0-16. This will represent the different lengths of stay.

Step 4. Plot a dot for each data element on the intersection of each category and length of stay.

Mean

The mean is the arithmetic average of all values in a group or population. It is symbolized as a "μ" in entire populations or a "$\bar{x}$" in sample populations. The way to compute the mean for a group is:

Step 1. Add all the values in the group

Step 2. Divide by the number of values in the group

EXAMPLE: Use data found in the case study and compute the mean (average) length of stay.

Step 1. 5+2+7+4+8+7+6+14+5+4+7+10+9+5+8+4+6+5+3+11+8+4+6+5 +6+5+7+6+4+9=190

Step 2. 190/30 = 6.333

EXERCISE: Use data found in the case study and compute the mean (average) length of stay for all cases which receive a 4 gm sodium diet.

Step 1.

Step 2.

Geometric Mean

The geometric mean is frequently used in medicine and epidemiology to describe the mean of diagnostic related groups. It is a logarithmic mean and is symbolized by a "GM" or "G." Geometric means are considered less sensitive to extreme variation in the group than arithmetic means. To compute the geometric mean you will:

Step 1.   Multiply together all the values in the group.

Step 2.   Compute the root of the product using the number of values in the set as the root.

EXAMPLE: Use data found in the case study and compute the geometric mean length of stay

Step 1.   5X2X7X4X8X7X6X14X5X4X7X10X9X5X8X4X6X5X3X11X8
X4X6X5X6X5X7X6X4X9= 1.14471×10^{23}

Step 2. $\sqrt[30]{1.14471 \times 10^{23}}$ = 5.86979

EXERCISE: Use data found in the case study and compute the geometric mean length of stay for all cases which receive a 4 gm sodium diet.

Step 1.

Step 2.

Median

The median is the middle value in a group which contains an odd number of values. If the group contains an even number of values, the median is defined as the average of the two middle values. The median is used frequently in run charts as a benchmark value. Although there is no conventional symbol for it, an "M" or "Md" is sometimes used. To compute the median for a group you will:

Step 1.   Order all the values from least to most (or vice versa).

Step 2.   Find the middle value; half of the values will be larger and half will be smaller than this amount.

Step 3.   If there are an even number of values in the group, compute the mean of the middle two values.

EXAMPLE: Using the data found in the case study determine the median for the length of stay.

    Step 1.   2,3,4,4,4,4,4,5,5,5,5,5,5,6,6,6,6,6,7,7,7,7,8,8,8,9,9,10,11,14

    Step 2.   6,6

    Step 3.   6

EXERCISE: Using the data found in the case study determine the median length of stay for the cases which receive a 4 gm sodium diet.

    Step 1.

    Step 2.

    Step 3.

Mode

    The mode is the most frequently occurring ("most popular") value in a given group. Clinicians can use this value while developing critical pathways to demonstrate the most popular forms of treatments or the most common patient outcomes. To compute the mode of a population, you will:

    Step 1.   Count the number of incidents of each value in the group.

    Step 2.   Select the most frequently occurring value; if there is a tie for the most frequent value, they are both considered the mode.

    Step 3.   Select the mode.

EXAMPLE: Using the data in the case study, determine the mode of the length of stay.

Step 1. LOS Groups	Step 2. Number of Values
2 Days	1
3 Days	1
4 Days	5
5 Days	6
6 Days	5
7 Days	4
8 Days	3
9 Days	2
10 Days	1

Step 1. LOS Groups	Step 2. Number of Values
11 Days	1
14 Days	1

Step 3.   Mode = 5 Days

TABLE 4. Central Tendency Test Summary

STATISTICAL TEST	FORMULA	RECOMMENDED DATA PRESENTATION
Mean	$\dfrac{x_1 + x_2 + x_3 + x_n}{n}$	Table, histogram, bar graph
Geometric Mean	$\sqrt[n]{x_1 \times x_2 \times x_3 \times x_n}$	Table, histogram, bar graph
Median	The middle number in a set after they are placed in ascending or descending order.	Table, central tendency in run chart, histogram, bar graph
Mode	The most frequently occurring value in a set of numbers.	Table, histogram, bar graph

Measures of Variation

Even though central tendency computations start to describe the target population, they do not give the whole picture. Range and standard deviation are common measures of variations and describe the amount of diversity within a given population.

Range

The most elementary measure of variation is the range. The range is the difference between the largest and smallest values in a group. The purpose of the range is to illustrate wide variances in values. Clinicians can use range to determine if there are variations in practice or patient outcomes. The larger the range, the greater the variation among members of the group. To compute the range for a population, simply:

Step 1.   Rank all values from smallest to largest.

Step 2.   Subtract the smallest value from the largest value.

EXAMPLE: Using the data in the case study, determine the range of the lengths of stay.

Step 1.   2,3,4,4,4,4,4,5,5,5,5,5,5,6,6,6,6,6,7,7,7,7,8,8,8,9,9,10,11,14

Step 2.   14 - 2 = 12

EXERCISE: Using the data in the case study, determine the range of the lengths of stay for cases which received Loop diuretics on Day one.

Step 1.

Step 2.

Standard Deviation

Standard deviation is the most common measurement of variation used for analyzing health care data. It is defined as the positive square root of the variance and measures the spread of data about the mean. To make the standard deviation meaningful, clinicians need to know the mean for the group.

To compute the standard deviation $\sigma = \sqrt{\dfrac{\sum (x - \bar{x})^2}{n - 1}}$, you will:

Step 1.   Compute the mean for the group.

Step 2.   Subtract the mean from each value to form the deviation.

Step 3.   Square each deviation.

Step 4.   Add the squared deviations together.

Step 5.   Subtract 1 from the number of values in the group.

Step 6.   Divide the sum of the squared deviation in step 4 by the difference obtained in step 5 (This is the variance).

Step 7.   Take the square root of the variance in step 6.

EXAMPLE: Using the case study information, determine the length of stay standard deviation for all patients who received a 2 gm sodium diet.

Step 1.   5+8+4+10+4+6+3+8+4+5+6= 63/11 = 5.73

Step 2.   Subtract the mean from each value to form the deviation.

Step 3.   Square each deviation.

Step 4.   Add the squared deviations together.

Patient	Length of Stay	Avg. Length of Stay	Deviation	Squared Deviation
1	5	-5.73	= -.73	0.5329
5	8	-5.73	= 2.27	+5.1529
10	4	-5.73	= -1.73	+2.9929
12	10	-5.73	= 4.27	+18.2329
16	4	-5.73	= -1.73	+2.9929
17	6	-5.73	= .27	+0.0729
19	3	-5.73	= -2.73	+7.4529
21	8	-5.73	= 2.27	+5.1529
22	4	-5.73	= -1.73	+2.9929
24	5	-5.73	= .73	+0.5329
28	6	-5.73	= .27	+0.0729
TOTAL				=46.1819

Step 5.   11 - 1 =10

Step 6.   46.1819 / 10 = 4.61819 (This is the variance)

Step 7. $\sqrt{4.61819}$ = 2.1489974 or 2.15

EXAMPLE: Using the case study information, determine the standard deviation for length of stay using all patients who were not weighed

Step 1.

Step 2.   Subtract the mean from each value to form the deviation.

Step 3.   Square each deviation.

Step 4.   Add the squared deviations together.

Patient	Length of Stay	Avg. Length of Stay	Deviation	Squared Deviation
		-	=	
		-	=	+

Patient	Length of Stay	Avg. Length of Stay	Deviation	Squared Deviation
		-	=	+
		-	=	+
		-	=	+
		-	=	+
		-	=	+
		-	=	+
		-	=	+
		-	=	+
		-	=	+
		-	=	+
TOTAL				=

Step 5.   Df =

Step 6.   /   =   (This is the variance)

Step 7.   √‾‾‾‾‾   =

STATISTICAL TEST	FORMULA	RECOMMENDED DATA DISPLAY
Range	Largest value - smallest value	Footnote, table, x-axis for histograms and bar graphs
Standard Deviation	$\sigma = \sqrt{\dfrac{\sum (x - \bar{x})^2}{n-1}}$	Table, line graph, control charts limits

Measures of Nominal Data

Nominal data does not measure the actual counts or frequency of occurrences. Rather, it measures proportions, ratios and rates. These methods allow clinicians to describe clusters of data relative to the whole group. Proportions and rates can assist clinicians in describing the prevalence of an intervention or patient outcome.

Proportion and Percentage

A proportion is the number of cases with a specified characteristic or group of characteristics divided by the total number of cases in the group. Proportions are useful in determining the frequency of a particular occurrence.

Proportions are especially useful for analyzing patient incident reports, adverse drug reactions and patient complaints. A proportion can be converted into a percentage by simply multiplying it by 100. To determine a proportion, you would:

Step 1.   Divide the number of observations with a specific characteristic by the total number of observations (both with and without that characteristic).

Rate

A rate is similar to a proportion except it is multiplied by a base number and is computed for a specified period of time. The base number is usually 100, 1000, 10,000 or 100,000 and is selected so that the smallest proportion has at least one digit to the left of the decimal point. It is important to use the same base number when comparing one rate to another. Rates are generally used to present nosocomial infections. To determine a rate, clinicians will:

Step 1.   Divide the number of observations with a specific characteristic by the total number of observations within the specified time period.

Step 2.   Multiply the proportion by a constant base number.

STATISTICAL TEST	FORMULA	RECOMMENDED DATA DISPLAY
Proportion	$Proportion = \dfrac{a}{a+b}$	Pie chart, line graph
Percentage	$Percentage = \dfrac{a}{a+b} \times 100$	Pie chart, line graph, bar chart
Rate	$Rate = \dfrac{a}{a+b} \times k$	Line graph, bar chart, histogram

3

Inferential Statistics Made Simple

The previously presented statistical tests tell clinicians what the population looks like but not why or how they arrived at this point. The next group of statistical tests allows clinicians to test their established hypotheses by making comparisons among different populations and correlating the interventions with outcomes. These inferential statistics tests can be applied to the collected data to determine why and how an outcome occurred.

Certain concepts are pivotal in understanding inferential statistics. They are:

1. Probability

2. Rule of addition

3. Rule of multiplication

4. Significance level

5. Z-score

6. Confidence interval

By understanding these key concepts, clinicians will be better equipped to perform and interpret inferential statistical tests such as chi square, t-test, z-test, correlation coefficient and ANOVA.

Probability

Probability measures the likelihood that a specific event or outcome will occur. It is expressed as a ratio, which is computed by dividing the number of times a result occurs by the total number of cases. If the outcome is sure to occur, the probability is one (1); if the outcome cannot occur it is zero (0). Understanding probability is important because it is a basic principle used in chi square and fisher exact tests to show if a specific critical pathway outcome occurs by chance or as a result of a pathway.

To compute probability, clinicians will:

Step 1. Count the number of times an event occurs.

Step 2. Divide the number of times an event occurs by the total number of values in the group.

EXAMPLE: Using the data in the case study, determine the probability of a patient having a length of stay of six days.

Step 1. 6 Days = 5 cases

Step 2. 5/30 =.1666

EXERCISE: Using the data in the case study, determine the probability of a patient who was **not** weighed having a length of stay of six days.

Step 1.

Step 2.

Rule of Addition

The rule of addition is used to describe the probability of at least one mutually exclusive event occurring when two or more types of independent events are possible. To compute probability using the rule of addition, clinicians will:

Step 1. Compute the probability for each mutually exclusive group.

Step 2. Add all probabilities together.

EXAMPLE: Using the case study data, determine the probability for a patient developing either pulmonary edema **or** being discharged within four days.

Step 1. Pulmonary Edema: 4/30 =.133 Discharged within four days: 7/30 =.233

Step 2. .133 +.233 =.366

EXERCISE: Using the case study data, determine the probability for eating a regular diet **or** being weighed at least once during this hospitalization.

      Step 1.

      Step 2.

Rule of Multiplication

      The rule of multiplication is used to determine the probability of two or more independent events all occurring. This is computed by multiplying all of the individual probabilities together. To perform this computation:

      Step 1.   Compute the probability for each independent event.

      Step 2.   Multiply together all probabilities from step 1.

EXAMPLE: Determine the probability of a patient having **both** pulmonary edema **and** having a 6 day length of stay.

      Step 1.   Pulmonary Edema: 4/30 =.133 6 Day length of stay: 5/30 =.167

      Step 2.   .133 X .167 = 0.0222

EXERCISE: Determine the probability of a patient having **both** pulmonary edema **and** being given a diuretic within 0-2 hours.

      Step 1.   Pulmonary Edema: Received diuretic within 0 - 2 hrs:

      Step 2.   X   =

Level of Significance

      Level of significance is the probability of observing a test result equal to or more extreme than the event can actually be observed from chance alone. This probability is represented by the letter p (for probability) and is a number between zero (0) and one (1). The smaller the significance level the more stringent the test. The significance level is established in advance of the test and is sometimes referred to as a **critical test value** or **alpha level.** Commonly used significance levels are 0.05 (1 chance in 20), 0.01 (1 chance in 100), or 0.001 (1 chance in 1,000).

      For example, clinicians may establish a critical value of .05 for determining if a particular treatment reduces length of stay by at least one day. When collecting data on the use of vasodilators, clinicians found that congestive heart failure patients using vasodilators had a probability value of .02. Comparing a p-value of .02 to the critical value of .05 shows that the probability of reducing the length of stay by pure chance is less likely than the critical value established before the test began.

It is important to understand significance level because statistical tests such as t-tests, z-tests, chi square and Fisher exact tests use the significance level to decide whether to accept or reject the null hypothesis.

Z-Score

The **z-score expresses the deviation from the mean in standard deviation units and is synonymous with terms such as z transformation, a standard score or a critical ratio.** Z-score is based on the **Central Limit Theorem,** a rule stating that the sampling distribution of means from any population will be normal for large samples. Converting actual values to z-score allows clinicians to use the area of the

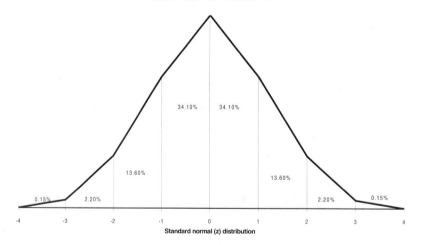

Normal Gaussian Distribution

normal distribution curve to determine the probability of occurrence for a given value. To compute the z-score, $z = \frac{x - \bar{x}}{\sigma}$, clinicians will:

Step 1.   Compute the mean for the group.

Step 2.   Compute standard deviation.

Step 3.   Subtract the mean from the designated value.

Step 4.   Divide the answer from step 3 by the standard deviation.

EXAMPLE: Using the case study data, determine the z-score for the length of stay of six days.

        Step 1.   Mean = 6.333

        Step 2.   SD =2.54

        Step 3.   6- 6.33 = -.33

        Step 4.   -.33/2.54 = -.13

        Step 5.   Mark on the graph below where the length of stay falls as a z-score.

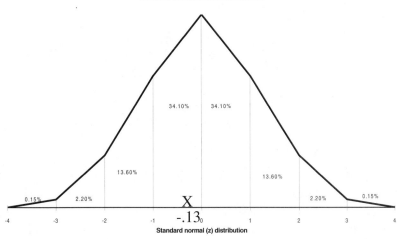

Normal Gaussian Distribution

34.10%   34.10%

13.60%   13.60%

0.15%   2.20%   2.20%   0.15%

X

$-.13_0$

-4   -3   -2   -1   1   2   3   4

Standard normal (z) distribution

EXERCISE: Using the patients who received a vasodilator, determine the z-score for the length of stay of six days.

        Step 1.   Mean =

        Step 2.   SD =

        Step 3.

        Step 4.

Step 5.   Mark on the graph below where the z-score is located.

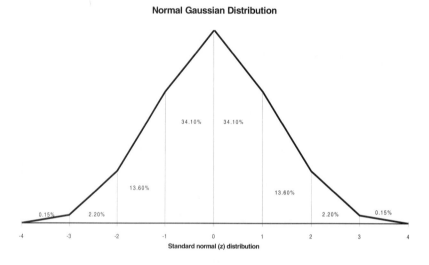

Normal Gaussian Distribution

Confidence Intervals

Confidence Interval (CI) is the range of values having a given probability of containing an unknown sample parameter (mean or proportion) given a specific significance level. Common Confidence Intervals are 90 percent, 95 percent and 99 percent. The boundaries are called Confidence Limits and are the values having a given probability that the unknown parameter is located between them. To express Confidence Intervals and Confidence Limits a clinicians might state "There is a 95 percent chance that the average length of stay for patients with congestive heart failure will be between four to 10 days."

STATISTICAL TEST	FORMULA	RECOMMENDED DATA DISPLAY
Probability	$P = \dfrac{n_a}{n}$	Table, footnote
Rule of Addition	P(A or B) = P(A) + P(B)	Table, footnote
Rule of Multiplication	P(A and B) = P(A) x P(B)	Table, footnote
Z-score	$z = \dfrac{x - \mu}{\sigma}$	Not applicable

Chi Square

The most commonly used statistical test for comparing frequency or proportions of two or more independent groups is chi square. Chi square is used to test the null hypothesis by determining the probability of a difference occurring between the groups by chance alone. It is also used to test the dependent relationship between the process variables within each group. To perform a chi square test, each group involved must be mutually exclusive and the expected frequency for each group must be equal to or greater than two.

In health care, chi square is used to show that a specific set of clinical interventions impacts a patient or financial outcome. For example, the length of stay for pneumonia patients may have a dependent relationship on the type of antibiotic used.

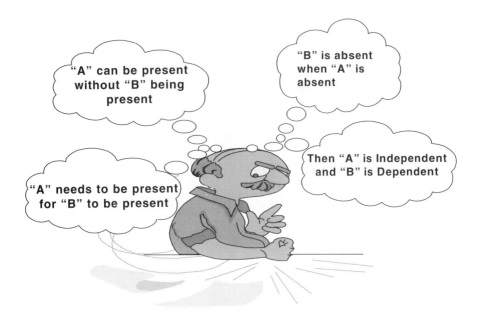

To interpret a chi square test, $x^2(df) = \sum\limits_{\substack{All \\ Cells}} \frac{(o-e)^2}{e}$ clinicians can use a chi square critical value chart. An abbreviated critical value chart is shown on the next page.

Degree of Freedom	Level of Significance			
	0.10	0.05	0.01	0.001
1	2.706	3.841	6.635	10.828
2	4.605	5.991	9.210	13.816
3	6.251	7.815	11.345	16.266
4	7.779	9.488	13.277	18.467
5	9.236	11.071	15.086	20.515

To perform a chi square test, clinicians follow these procedures:

Step 1. Formulate a null and alternative hypothesis about the relationship between a treatment modality and the patient outcome.

Step 2. Select the desired level of significance.

Step 3. Compute the degree of freedom for the test.df = (# of rows - 1) X (# of columns - 1).

Step 4. Label each column with dependent outcomes and column for total.

Step 5. Label each row with processes variables and a row for total.

Step 6. Place frequencies in the table for each event.

Step 7. Add all frequencies found in the rows and place in the total column.

Step 8. Add all frequencies found in the columns and place in the total row.

Step 9. Compute the expected probability for each cell by multiplying the row total by the column total and dividing by the grand total.

Step 10. Subtract the expected frequency from the actual frequency.

Step 11. Square the difference between the observed and the expected frequencies for each cell.

Step 12. Divide the squared value of each cell in step 11 by the expected value for the cell.

Step 13. Add all the quotients together.

Step 14.   The critical value is the number located where the degree of
freedom row intersects with the level of significance column; if the
sum is greater than the critical value the null hypothesis is rejected.

EXAMPLE: Determine if there is a relationship between receiving a 2 gm sodium
diet and having a length of stay of less than five days.

Step 1.   **Null Hypothesis:** Patients with congestive heart failure who
receive a 2 gm sodium diet **do not** have a greater possibility of
being discharged from the hospital by day five.
Alternative Hypothesis: Patients with congestive heart failure who
receive a 2 gm sodium diet have a greater possibility of being
discharged by day five.

Step 2.   Significance level for chi square will be 0.05.

Step 3.   Degree of freedom: (2 -1) X (2 -1) = 1.

Steps 4-8	Cases with a length of stay of five days or less	Cases with a length of stay of six days or more	Total # of cases
Cases with 2 GM sodium diet	6	5	11
Cases without 2 GM sodium diet	7	12	19
Total # of cases	13	17	30

Step 4.   See column headings.

Step 5.   See row headings.

Step 6.   Place frequency of each category of cases in corresponding table
cells.

Step 7.   Add rows.

Step 8.   Add columns.

Step 9. Compute expected frequencies for each cell: Rule of Multiplication.

Step 9	Cases with a length of stay of five days or less	Cases with a length of stay of six days or more	Total # of cases
Cases with 2 GM sodium diet	$\frac{11}{30} \times \frac{13}{30} = 0.1548$ $0.1548 \times 30 = 4.7$	$\frac{11}{30} \times \frac{17}{30} = 0.204$ $0.204 \times 30 = 6.23$	11
Cases without 2 GM sodium diet	$\frac{19}{30} \times \frac{13}{30} = 0.274$ $0.274 \times 30 = 8.23$	$\frac{17}{30} \times \frac{19}{30} = 0.36$ $0.36 \times 30 = 10.77$	19
Total # of cases	13	17	30

Step 10. Subtract the expected frequency from the actual.

Step 10	Cases with a length of stay of five days or less	Cases with a length of stay of six days or more	Total # of cases
Cases with 2 GM sodium diet	6 - 4.77 = 1.23	5 - 6.23 = -1.23	11
Cases without 2 GM sodium diet	7 - 8.23 = -1.23	12 - 10.77 = 1.23	19
Total # of cases	13	17	30

Step 11. Square the difference between the observed and the expected frequencies for each cell.

Step 11	Cases with a length of stay of five days or less	Cases with a length of stay of six days or more	Total # of cases
Cases with 2 GM sodium diet	1.5129	1.5129	11
Cases without 2 GM sodium diet	1.5129	1.5129	19
Total # of cases	13	17	30

Step 12. Divide the squared value of each cell in step 11 by the expected value for the cell.

Step 12	Cases with a length of stay of five days or less	Cases with a length of stay of six days or more	Total # of cases
Cases with 2 GM sodium diet	1.5129/ 4.77 =.317	1.5129/ 6.23 =.245	11
Cases without 2 GM sodium diet	1.5129/ 8.23 =.184	1.5129/ 10.77 = 0.140	19
Total # of cases	13	17	30

Step 13. .317 + .245 +.184 + .140 =.886

Step 14. (Critical value = 3.841) The null hypothesis is not rejected.

EXERCISE: Determine if there is a relationship between a patient being weighed (even one time) and having a length of stay of less than five days.

Step 1. **Null Hypothesis:**
Alternative Hypothesis:

Step 2. Significance level for chi square will be 0.05

Step 3. Degree of freedom: (   ) X (   ) =

Steps 4-8			Total # of cases
Total # of cases			

Step 4. Set column headings.

Step 5. Set row headings.

Step 6. Place frequency of each category of cases in corresponding table cells.

Step 7. Add rows.

Step 8. Add columns.

Step 9. Compute expected frequencies for each cell: Rule of Multiplication.

Step 9			Total # of cases
Total # of cases			

Step 10. Subtract the expected frequency from the actual.

Step 10			Total # of cases
Total # of cases			

Step 11. Square the difference between the observed and the expected frequencies each cell.

Step 11			Total # of cases

Step 11			Total # of cases
Total # of cases			

Step 12. Divide the squared value of each cell in step 11 by the expected value for the cell.

Step 12			Total # of cases
Total # of cases	.		

Step 13.　　　+　　　+　　　+　　　=

Step 14.　(Critical value =　　　) The null hypothesis is

T-Test

T-tests are used to compare the mean of one group with either a standard or with the mean of another group. **The purpose of this comparison is to determine the probability of getting this magnitude of difference by chance alone.** Stated another way, t-tests are used to determine if there is a significant difference between groups. For example, there might by a difference between congestive heart failure cases using ACE inhibitors and those not using ACE inhibitors. However, the difference between the cases is only an average of 0.1 minute. This difference is not significant enough to warrant changing all practice. In general the larger the difference between the two means, the more likely it is that the t-test will be significant. However, there are two other factors which influence this significance, variability and sample size. Given the same mean difference, groups with less variability will be more likely to be significantly different than groups with wide variability. Variability is based on the **standard error of the mean** and is calculated by dividing the variance (which is the square of the standard deviation) by the sample size.

There are several guidelines which should be considered when using the t-test. These are:

- The independent variable needs to be a nominal variable (a number).

- Two groups are needed for comparison (More than two groups normally requires an ANOVA test to determine if there is a difference among groups).

- The dependent variable should be interval or ratio level, although ordinal-level data can be treated as interval level data.

To interpret t-test results, clinicians need to be aware of whether they are testing a directional hypothesis or a non-directional hypothesis. A directional hypothesis uses a one tailed test to interpret the results and is considered a more powerful test, because the value yielded by the statistical test does not have to be so large to be significant at a given level.

To use a one-tailed test of significance, however, a sound theoretical basis for the directional hypothesis is needed. It cannot be based on a hunch.

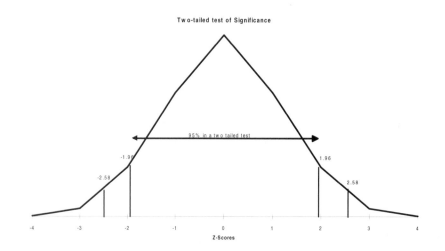

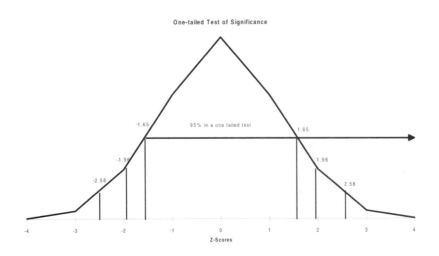

One-tailed Test of Significance

A concept which needs to be understood about t-tests is the difference between conducting a one and two tail analysis. A one tail t-test is used when the hypothesis states the anticipated direction of the difference.

For example, testing the average length of stay for patients eating a 2 gm sodium diet will be at one day less than patients not on a 2 gm sodium diet. A two tail t-test is used when the direction of the difference is unknown.

There are several types of t-tests, these include a basic (pooled) t-test, a separate t-test and a correlated or paired t-test. The **basic t-test** is appropriate when the variances of the two groups are equal. The **separate t-test** is used when a more conservative formula is required because the variances for the two groups are not the same. If the two groups being compared are matched or paired on some basis then a **paired or correlated t-test** is appropriate.

There are four assumptions underlying the t-test. These assumptions are:

- First, the t-test requires at least interval-level data for the dependent measure

- Each subject will contribute one score to the distribution of one specific group

- The distribution of the dependent measure is normal

- The groups are similar in their variances (homogeneity of variance)

To perform this test, the sample must have normal distribution. Two strengths of the t-test are the ability to test:

1. Small sample sizes (less than 30 cases)

2. When the standard deviation is unknown

Degree	Area in 1 Tail				
of	0.05	0.025	0.01	0.005	0.0005
Freedom	Area in 2 Tails				
	0.10	0.05	0.02	0.01	0.001
1	3.078	6.314	31.82	63.66	636.62
2	1.886	2.920	6.965	9.925	22.33
3	1.638	2.353	4.541	5.841	10.21
4	1.533	2.132	3.747	4.604	7.173
5	1.476	2.015	3.365	4.032	5.893
6	1.440	1.943	3.143	3.707	5.208
7	1.415	1.895	2.998	3.499	4.785
8	1.397	1.860	2.896	3.355	4.501
9	1.383	1.833	2.821	3.250	4.297
10	1.372	1.812	2.764	3.169	4.144
11	1.363	1.796	2.718	3.106	4.025
12	1.356	1.782	2.681	3.055	3.930
13	1.350	1.771	2.650	3.012	3.852
14	1.345	1.761	2.624	2.977	3.787
15	1.341	1.753	2.602	2.947	3.733
16	1.337	1.746	2.583	2.921	3.686
17	1.333	1.740	2.567	2.898	3.646
18	1.330	1.734	2.552	2.878	3.611
19	1.328	1.729	2.539	2.861	3.579
20	1.325	1.725	2.528	2.845	3.552
21	1.323	1.721	2.518	2.831	3.527
22	1.321	1.717	2.508	2.819	3.505
23	1.319	1.714	2.500	2.807	3.485

Degree	Area in 1 Tail				
of	0.05	0.025	0.01	0.005	0.0005
Freedom	Area in 2 Tails				
	0.10	0.05	0.02	0.01	0.001
24	1.318	1.711	2.492	2.797	3.467
25	1.316	1.708	2.485	2.787	3.450
26	1.315	1.706	2.479	2.779	3.435
27	1.314	1.703	2.473	2.771	3.421
28	1.313	1.701	2.467	2.763	3.408
29	1.311	1.699	2.462	2.756	3.396
30	1.310	1.697	2.457	2.750	3.385

To compute a separate t-test clinicians will use the following formula, $t = \dfrac{\bar{x}_1 - \bar{x}_2}{\sqrt{\dfrac{s_1^2}{n_1} + \dfrac{s_2^2}{n_2}}}$:

Step 1.   State the null and alternative hypothesis about the difference between the two populations.

Step 2.   Select an alpha level for the test.

Step 3.   Calculate the df = n - 2.

Step 4.   Compute the sample mean for the first group.

Step 5.   Compute the sample mean for the second group.

Step 6.   Compute the first group variance (σ^2).

Step 7.   Compute the second group variance (σ^2).

Step 8.   Subtract the answer for step 5 from the answer of step 4.

Step 9.   Divide the variance of the first group by the number of cases in the first sample.

Step 10.   Divide the variance of the second group by the number of cases in the second sample.

Step 11.   Sum the answers of step 9 and 10.

Step 12.   Compute the square root of the answer to step 11.

Step 13.   Compute the quotient of step 8 divided by the answer of step 12.

Step 14.   Compare the answer from step 13 with the critical value selected in step 2; if the t-test value is higher than the critical value, the null hypothesis can be rejected.

EXAMPLE: Clinicians wanted to determine with 95 percent accuracy if the average length of the stay for patients who receive a vasodilator is significantly less than those patients who do not receive a vasodilator.

Step 1.   Null hypothesis: The use of vasodilators does not decrease the length of stay of patients with congestive heart failure.

Alternative hypothesis: The use of vasodilators decreases the length of stay of patients with congestive heart failure.

Step 2.   Alpha level = 0.05

Step 3.   df = 30 - 2 = 28

Step 4. $\bar{x} = \dfrac{5+4+6+14+4+8+11+4+6+6+6+9}{12} = 6.92$ (group without vasodilators)

Step 5. $\dfrac{2+7+8+7+5+7+10+9+5+4+6+5+3+8+5+5+7+4}{18} = 5.94$ (group with vasodilators)

Step 6. $\sigma^2 = 3.09^2 = 9.5481$

Step 7. $\sigma^2 = 2.09^2 = 4.3681$

Step 8.   6.92 - 5.94 = 0.98

Step 9.   9.5481/ 12 = 0.795675

Step 10.   4.3681 / 18 = 0.2426722

Step 11.   0.795675 + 0.2426722 = 1.0383472

Step 12. $\sqrt{1.0383472} = 1.0189932$

Step 13.   0.98 / 1.0189932 = 0.96

Step 14.   critical value = 1.31

0.96 < 1.31: The null hypothesis can not be rejected

Correlation Coefficient

The Pearson Product Moment Correlation Coefficient is a measure of the degree to which two variables are linearly related. This means there is an interdependency between clinical interventions and a patient outcome. **Correlation coefficient is used only when both the clinical intervention and the outcome measurement is an ordinal scale number.** Examples of this type of clinical interventions are the timing of an intervention, the number of chest x-rays and the average daily dose for a medication. Examples of clinical outcomes which are appropriate for correlation coefficient is the length of stay in days, number of complications or cost of care.

The result of a correlation coefficient is either positive or negative and ranges in value between -1 and 1. A positive correlation indicates that an increase in one variable will correspond to an increase in the other variable. A negative correlation indicates that as one variable increases the other variable decreases. To compute a Correlation Coefficient, the mean of both variable groups must be known. Clinicians should follow this procedure:

Step 1.   Compute the mean for the first variable (x).

Step 2.   Compute the mean for the second variable (y).

Step 3.   Arrange the variables in corresponding rows in a table.

Step 4.   Subtract the answer from step 1 from each of the values in the first group of variables $(x - \bar{x})$.

Step 5.   Subtract the answer from step 2 from each of the values in the second group of variables $(y - \bar{y})$.

Step 6.   Multiply the results of step 4 by corresponding results from step 5.

Step 7.   Add together all the products from step 6.

Step 8.   Square each difference computed in step 4.

Step 9.   Add together each square computed in step 8.

Step 10. Square each difference computed in step 5.

Step 11. Add together each square computed in step 10.

Step 12. Compute the square root of the sum found in step 9.

Step 13. Compute the square root of the sum found in step 11.

Step 14. Multiply the square root found in step 12 by the square root found in step 13.

Step 15. Divide the result from step 7 by the product of step 14.

Step 16. Determine the correlation between variables using Colton's rule of thumb shown below.

Correlation values	Degree of relationship
0 to 0.25 or 0 to -0.25	Little if any
.26 to 0.49 or -0.26 to -0.49	Low
0.50 to 0.69 or -0.50 to -0.69	Moderate
0.70 to 0.89 or -0.70 to - 0.89	High
0.90 to 1.00 or - 0.90 to - 1.00	Very high

EXAMPLE: Using the second case study, determine if there is a correlation between the initial timing of antibiotic administration and the length of stay.

Step 1. 2+6+1+8+2+10+4+2+12+3+5+4+5+2+6+3+1+.5+8+4+3+24+6+8 +3+4+4+5+2+3 = 150.5/30 = 5.02 (hrs)

Step 2. 5+7+4+6+5+9+7+4+5+6+6+5+4+4+4+4+3+3+10+6+5+10+5+6+ 4+7+5+8+5+6= 168/ 30 = 5.6 (days)

Step 3. Arrange variables in corresponding rows in a table (See table below).

Step 4. Subtract the answer from step 1 from each of the values in the first group of variables $(x - \bar{x})$.

Step 5. Subtract the answer from step 2 from each of the values in the second group of variables $(y - \bar{y})$.

Step 6. Multiply the results of step 4 by corresponding results from step 5.

Step 7. Add together all the products from step 6.

Step 8. Square each difference computed in step 4.

Step 9. Add together each square computed in step 8.

Step 10. Square each difference computed in step 5.

Step 11. Add together each square computed in step 10 .

Pa-tient	x	y	Step 4 $x - \bar{x}$	Step 5 $y - \bar{y}$	Step 6 $(x - \bar{x})(y - \bar{y})$	Step 8 $(x - \bar{x})^2$	Step 10 $(y - \bar{y})^2$
1	2	5	-3.02	-0.6	1.812	9.1204	0.36
2	6	7	0.98	1.4	1.372	0.9604	1.96
3	1	4	-4.02	-1.6	6.432	16.1604	2.56
4	8	6	2.98	0.4	1.192	8.8804	0.16
5	2	5	-3.02	-0.6	1.812	9.12.4	0.36
6	1 0	9	4.98	3.4	16.932	24.8004	11.56
7	4	7	-1.02	1.4	-1.428	1.0404	1.96
8	2	4	-3.02	-1.6	4.832	9.1204	2.56
9	1 2	5	6.98	-0.6	-4.188	48.7204	0.36
10	3	6	-2.02	0.4	-0.808	4.0804	0.16
11	5	6	-0.02	0.4	-0.008	0.0004	0.16
12	4	5	-1.02	-0.6	0.612	1.0404	0.36
13	5	4	-0.02	-1.6	0.032	0.0004	2.56
14	2	4	-3.02	-1.6	4.832	9.1204	2.56
15	6	4	0.98	-1.6	-1.568	0.9604	2.56
16	3	4	-2.02	-1.6	3.232	4.0804	2.56
17	1	3	-4.02	-2.6	10.452	16.1604	6.76
18	. 5	3	-4.52	-2.6	11.752	20.4304	6.76
19	8	1 0	2.98	4.4	13.112	8.8804	19.36
20	4	6	-1.02	0.4	-0.408	1.0404	0.16
21	3	5	-2.02	-0.6	1.212	4.0804	0.36
22	2 4	1 0	18.98	4.4	83.512	360.2404	19.36
23	6	5	0.98	-0.6	-0.588	0.9604	0.36
24	8	6	2.98	0.4	1.192	8.8804	0.16
25	3	4	-2.02	-1.6	3.232	4.0804	2.56
26	4	7	-1.02	1.4	-1.428	1.0404	1.96
27	4	5	-1.02	-0.6	0.612	1.040	0.36
28	5	8	-0.02	2.4	-0.048	0.0004	5.76
29	2	5	-3.02	-0.6	1.812	9.12	0.36

Pa-tient	x	y	Step 4 $x - \bar{x}$	Step 5 $y - \bar{y}$	Step 6 $(x - \bar{x})(y - \bar{y})$	Step 8 $(x - \bar{x})^2$	Step 10 $(y - \bar{y})^2$
30	3	6	-2.02	0.4	-0.808	4.0804	0.16
Sum					Step 7: 158.7	Step 9: 587.242	Step 11: 97.2

Step 12. Compute the square root of the sum found in Step 9: 24.233077

Step 13. Compute the square root of the sum found in Step 11: 9.859006

Step 14. 24.233077 X 9.859006 = 238.91405

Step 15. 158.7 / 238.91405 = 0.6642556

Step 16. Step 16. 0.6642556 = Moderate correlation

EXERCISE: Using the second case study, determine if there is a correlation between the number of chest x-rays and the length of stay.

Step 1.

Step 2.

Step 3. Arrange variables in corresponding rows in a table (See table below).

Step 4. Subtract the answer from step 1 from each of the values in the first group of variables $(x - \bar{x})$.

Step 5. Subtract the answer from step 2 from each of the values in the second group of variables $(y - \bar{y})$.

Step 6. Multiply the results of step 4 by corresponding results from step 5.

Step 7. Add together all the products from step 6.

Step 8. Square each difference computed in step 4.

Step 9. Add together each square computed in step 8.

Step 10. Square each difference computed in step 5.

Step 11. Add together each square computed in step 10.

Patient	x	y	Step 4 $x - \bar{x}$	Step 5 $y - \bar{y}$	Step 6 $(x - \bar{x})(y - \bar{y})$	Step 8 $(x - \bar{x})^2$	Step 10 $(y - \bar{y})^2$
1							
2							
3							

Patient	x	y	Step 4 $x - \bar{x}$	Step 5 $y - \bar{y}$	Step 6 $(x - \bar{x})(y - \bar{y})$	Step 8 $(x - \bar{x})^2$	Step 10 $(y - \bar{y})^2$
4							
5							
6							
7							
8							
9							
10							
11							
12							
13							
14							
15							
16							
17							
18							
19							
20							
21							
22							
23							
24							
25							
26							
27							
28							
29							
30							
Sum					Step 7:	Step 9:	Step 11:

Step 12.   Compute the square root of the sum found in step 9:

Step 13.   Compute the square root of the sum found in step 11:

Step 14.   X   =

Step 15.   /   =
Step 16.   =

ANOVA: Analysis of Variance

Many times, a clinician wants to compare several groups on a particular measure. For example, a question may arise whether the type of antibiotic impacts the length of stay. Because there are more than two classes of antibiotics a t-test is not appropriate. To conduct a series of t-tests to compare each group with all other groups would cause the rate of error to increase exponentially by the number of tests conducted. To avoid the risk of incorrectly rejecting the null hypothesis, clinicians can examine the differences among the groups through an analysis that considers the variation across all groups at once. This test is the Analysis of Variance (ANOVA).

The question answered by the ANOVA test is whether group means differ from each other. However, the ANOVA results may only indicate differences among the groups but do not tell which pairs of groups were different. To ascertain where the difference occurred, additional comparison analysis must be performed, such as a MANOVA or ANCOVA.

Data required to conduct an ANOVA is a nominal independent variable(s) which has two or more levels. This independent variable is called a factor. There are several types of ANOVAs.

- A one way ANOVA means that there is only one independent variable which is called a factor; gender is an example of a variable with two levels.

- A two-way ANOVA indicates two independent variables.

- A n-way ANOVA indicates the number of independent variables is defined by n. The dependent variable or outcome should be an interval or ratio level.

There are four basic assumptions made when conducting an ANOVA test:

- The dependent variable should be measured at the interval or ratio level.

- The groups should be mutually exclusive (independent of each other).

- The dependent variable should be normally distributed.

- The groups should have equal variances (homogeneity of variance requirements).

The statistical question using ANOVA is based on the null hypothesis: the assumption that all groups are equal and drawn from the same population. Any difference comes from a random sampling difference. Any variability of scores can be seen in two ways: First, the scores vary from each other in their own group; second, the groups vary from each other. The first variation is called within-group variation; the second variation is called between-group variation. Together the two types of variation add up to total variation.

Source of Variation	Sum of Squares	Degrees of Freedom	Mean Squares	F Ratio
Among groups	$SS_A = \sum n_j \bar{x}_j^2 - \dfrac{\left(\sum x_{ij}\right)^2}{N}$	$k-1$	$MS_A = \dfrac{SS_A}{k-1}$	$F = \dfrac{MS_A}{MS_E}$
Error	$SS_E = SS_T - SS_A$	$N-k$	$MS_E = \dfrac{SS_E}{N-k}$	
Total	$SS_T = \sum x^2_{ij} - \dfrac{\left(\sum x_{ij}\right)^2}{N}$	$N-1$		

To compute a one-way ANOVA:

Step 1. Formulate a null and alternate hypothesis.

Step 2. Select the desired critical value.

Step 3. Compute the mean of the first group.

Step 4. Compute the mean of the second group.

Step 5. Multiply the number of values in group one by the answer in step 3.

Step 6. Multiply the number of values in the second group by the value in step 4.

Step 7. Add the product of step and 5 and step 6.

Step 8. Divide the answer to step 7 by the sum of all values.

Step 9. Subtract the answer in step 8 from the mean of the first group found in step 3.

Step 10. Square the answer in step 9.

Step 11. Multiply the answer in step 10 by the number of values in the first group.

Step 12. Subtract the answer in step 8 from the mean of the second group found in step 4.

Step 13. Square the answer in step 12.

Step 14. Multiply the answer in step 13 by the number of values in the second group.

Step 15. Sum the answers in step 11 and step 14.

Step 16. Subtract 1 from the total number of groups in the test (in this case 2 - 1= 1).

Step 17. Divide the answer in step 15 by the answer in step 16. **This is the value of MS$_A$.**

To Compute the MS$_E$

Step 18. Subtract 1 from the total number of values in the first group.

Step 19. Subtract 1 from the total number of values in the second group.

Step 20. Sum the results of step 18 and step 19.

Step 21. Compute the standard deviation for the first group.

Step 22. Square the standard deviation for the first group (This is the variance).

Step 23. Multiply the result of step 18 by the answer to step 22.

Step 24. Compute the standard deviation for the second group.

Step 25. Square the answer in step 24 to find the variance.

Step 26. Multiply the result of step 19 by the answer to step 25.

Step 27. Sum the answers in step 23 and step 26.

Step 28. Divide the answer to step 27 by answer in step 20. **This is the Error mean Square or MS$_E$.**

Finally, the F ratio is found by:

Step 29. Divide the answer to step 17 by the answer to Step 28.

Step 30. Compare the value found is step 29 with the critical value found in the following abbreviated f distribution table.

Step 31. Reject or Don't reject the Null hypothesis.

TABLE 5. Percentage points or critical values for the F distribution corresponding to areas of 0.05 and 0.01 under the upper tail of the distribution.

Degree of Freedom, Denominator	Area	Degrees of Freedom, Numerator			
		1	2	3	4
1	0.05	161.4	199.5	215.7	230.2
	0.01	2052	4999.5	5403	5764
2	0.05	18.51	19.00	19.16	19.25
	0.01	98.50	99.00	99.17	99.25
3	0.05	10.13	9.55	9.28	9.12
	0.01	34.12	30.82	29.46	28.71
4	0.05	7.71	6.94	6.59	6.39
	0.01	21.20	18.00	16.69	15.98
5	0.05	6.61	5.79	5.41	5.19
	0.01	16.26	13.27	12.06	11.39
6	0.05	5.90	5.14	4.76	4.54
	0.01	13.75	10.92	9.78	9.15
7	0.05	5.59	4.74	4.35	4.12
	0.01	12.25	9.55	8.45	7.85
8	0.05	5.32	4.46	4.07	3.84
	0.01	11.26	8.66	7.59	7.01
9	0.05	5.12	4.26	3.86	3.63
	0.01	10.56	8.02	6.99	6.42
10	0.05	4.96	4.10	3.71	3.48
	0.01	10.04	7.56	6.55	5.99
12	0.05	4.75	3.98	3.49	3.26
	0.01	9.33	6.93	5.95	5.41
15	0.05	4.54	3.68	3.29	3.06
	0.01	8.68	6.36	5.42	4.89
20	0.05	4.35	3.49	3.10	2.87
	0.01	8.10	5.85	4.94	4.43
24	0.05	4.26	3.40	3.01	2.78
	0.01	7.82	5.61	4.72	4.22

TABLE 5. Percentage points or critical values for the F distribution corresponding to areas of 0.05 and 0.01 under the upper tail of the distribution.

Degree of Freedom, Denominator	Area	Degrees of Freedom, Numerator			
		1	2	3	4
30	0.05	4.17	3.32	2.92	2.69
	0.01	7.56	5.39	4.51	4.02
40	0.05	4.08	3.23	2.84	2.61
	0.01	7.31	5.18	4.31	3.83
60	0.05	4.00	3.15	2.76	2.53
	0.01	7.08	4.98	4.13	3.65
120	0.05	3.92	3.07	2.68	2.45
	0.01	6.85	4.79	3.95	3.48
∞	0.05	3.84	3.00	2.60	2.37
	0.01	6.63	4.61	3.78	3.32

EXAMPLE: Using the data found in the next table, determine if there is a length of stay difference among the antibiotic classes.

TABLE 6. Antibiotic Classification Analysis

Type of Antibiotics	First Generation Cephalosporin	Third Generation Cephalosporin	Penicillins
Length of Stay	4	4	4
	5	8	5
	9	6	9
	10	3	7
	2	6	14
	10	5	3
	3	6	6
	7	7	7
	6	4	8
		3	
Number of Cases	9	10	9
Mean	6.22	5.2	7
Standard Deviation	2.99	1.69	3.24

Step 1. Null hypothesis: There is no difference among the average length of stay for each class of antibiotic.

Alternative Hypothesis: This is a difference among the average length of stay for each class of antibiotic.

Step 2. Critical value will be 0.05

Step 3. 4+5+9+10+2+10+3+7+6 = 56/9 = 6.222

Step 4. 4+8+6+3+6+5+6+7+4+3 = 52/10 = 5.2

Step 5. 4+5+9+7+14+3+6+7+8 = 63/9 = 7

Step 6. 9 X 6.22 = 55.998

Step 7. 10 X 5.2 = 52

Step 8. 9 X 7 = 63

Step 9. 55.998 + 52 + 63 = 170.998

Step 10.   170.998 / 28 = 6.11

Step 11.   6.22 - 6.11 =.11

Step 12. $.11^2 = 0.0121$

Step 13.   .01211X 9 = 0.10899

Step 14.   5.2 - 6.11 = -.91

Step 15. $-.91^2 = 0.8281$

Step 16.   0.8281 X 10 = 8.281

Step 17.   7-6.11 =.89

Step 18. $.89^2 = 0.7921$

Step 19.   0.7921 X 9 = 7.1289

Step 20.   0.10899 + 8.281 + 7.1289 = 15.5998

Step 21.   3 - 1= 2

Step 22.   15.5998/ 2 = 7.7998 **This is the value of MS_A.**

To Compute the MS_E

Step 23.   9 -1 = 8

Step 24.   10 - 1 = 9

Step 25.   9 - 1 = 8

Step 26.   8 + 9 + 8 = 25

Step 27.   2.99

Step 28. $2.99^2 = 8.94$

Step 29.   8 X 8.94 = 71.52

Step 30.   1.69

Step 31. $1.69^2 = 2.86$

Step 32.   2.86 X 9 = 25.70

Step 33.   3.24

Step 34. $3.24^2 = 10.5$

Step 35.   10.5 X 8 = 83.98

Step 36.   71.52 + 25.70 + 83.98 = 181.2

Step 37.   181.2 / 25 = 7.25 **This is the Error mean Square or MS_E.**

Finally, the F ratio is found by:

Step 38.   7.7998 / 7.25 = 1.0758

Step 39.   1.0758 < 3.40

Step 40.   Cannot Reject the Null hypothesis.

Source of Variation	Sum of Squares	Degrees of Freedom	Mean Squares	F Ratio
Among groups	15.5998	2	7.7998	1.0758
Error	181.2	25	7.25	
Total	196.7998	27		

4

Determining Fiscal Impact of Improvement

With increased awareness of health care costs and emphasis on "value added activities," clinicians need to be able to analyze available financial information. The reason for this skill is to:

- Determine the financial health of an organization
- Demonstrate the cost-benefit of quality initiatives
- Determine the financial impact of future clinical improvement

Determining Financial Health

One of the skills required of all managers in health care is a basic understanding of financial reports, such as cash flow statements, balance sheets and profit and loss statements. By being able to interpret these three reports, quality management professionals can assess the health of an organization.

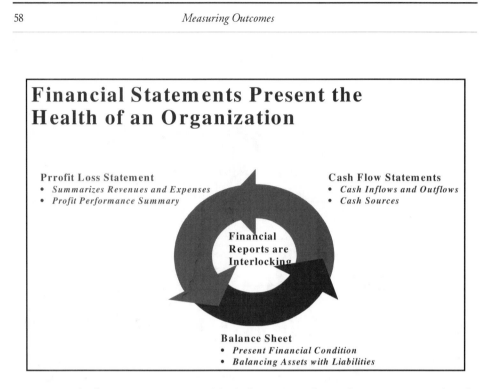

Financial Statements Present the Health of an Organization

Prrofit Loss Statement
- *Summarizes Revenues and Expenses*
- *Profit Performance Summary*

Cash Flow Statements
- *Cash Inflows and Outflows*
- *Cash Sources*

Financial Reports are Interlocking

Balance Sheet
- *Present Financial Condition*
- *Balancing Assets with Liabilities*

Cash flow statements provide information about the movement of cash, revenue sources and availability of cash. The profit and loss statement, also called an income statement, provides information about the profitability of an organization. The balance sheet presents a snapshot of the organization's financial condition at a given moment in time. The balance sheet lists all assets, including cash, accounts receivable, inventory, prepaid expenses, property, plant and equipment minus depreciation and all liabilities and equity.

Why is it important for clinicians and quality professionals to know about financial statements? Simply put, quality and resource initiatives impact the bottom line of health care organizations. For example, if an organization receives most of its revenue from indemnity insurance plans, then reducing the length of stay could negatively impact the bottom line of the organization.

By being aware of how the income statement is computed and the organization's case mix, quality management professionals can target quality and resource activities at areas which will be mutually beneficial for patients and the organization.

Income Statements Can Reflect Impact of Quality/Resource Initiatives

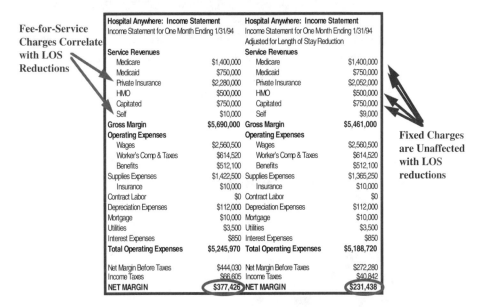

Fee-for-Service Charges Correlate with LOS Reductions

Fixed Charges are Unaffected with LOS reductions

Proving the Cost Benefit of Quality Initiatives

With growing emphasis on cost-containment and increasing pressure to prove "value added," many quality initiatives may be questioned in the future by administration and consumers regarding the benefits of making changes. Quality management professionals and clinicians will need to answer these questions with both qualitative and quantitative data.

Some of the main reasons for analyzing the financial costs and benefits of quality initiatives include:

- Determining if a quality initiative is cost-effective

- Identifying tangible benefits

- Determining return on investment

To ascertain the cost benefit of a particular quality or resource initiative, the net financial benefit needs to be calculated. This calculation consists of the difference between the financial benefits and the financial costs contributed to produce the improvement result.

Financial Benefits - Costs = Cost Benefit (Net Benefit)

To start this computation process, there needs to be a review of the organizational goals for quality initiatives. The organizational goal is the outcome measurement for supporting the quality initiative and will answer the question "Why should I support this effort?" Organizational goals are not limited to only patient outcomes or financial contributions but will include employee and market benefits.

Organizational Goals Gives Clues For Determining Cost-Benefits

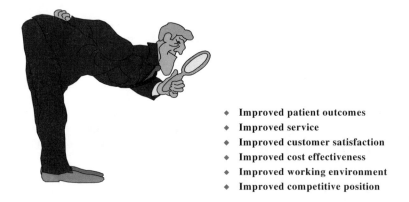

- Improved patient outcomes
- Improved service
- Improved customer satisfaction
- Improved cost effectiveness
- Improved working environment
- Improved competitive position

Once goals are selected for the quality initiative, the scope of costs and benefits included in the analysis should be determined. It is best to focus on short-term financial impact because these impacts are the easiest to defend and demonstrate a correlation with the quality improvement.

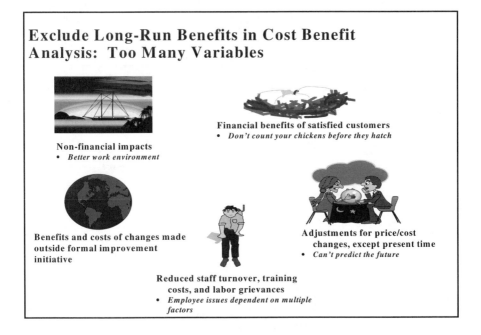

The guidelines for calculating cost benefits include selection of how cost and benefits will be measured. The two most common options are:

1. Measuring all costs and benefits

2. Using only marginal costs and benefits

To define financial terms used in the analysis:

- Specify inclusions and exclusions from calculations

- Determine the number of years for calculating the cost benefits

- Select a starting date for calculations

- Use present value of all centralized and project costs and benefits if initiatives cover multiple years

Terminology	Definition	Example
Financial Costs	Net marginal costs plus net revenue losses.	Reallocation of staff without experiencing an increase in payroll costs is $0.00 financial costs.
Financial Benefits	Net marginal cost savings plus net revenue increases.	If the cost of care for patients with bacterial pneumonia is decreased by $500.00 and the profit margin is increased by $200.00 then the financial benefit is $700.00 a patient.
Capital Cost Impact	Use depreciation rate as annual cost of all capital expenditures directly related to improvement.	A new computer system is purchased, depreciation is used as the capital cost impact.
Implementation Cost Impact	Length of training time X (Number of employees, physicians, etc. X cost of employees time) Only additional time worked will be included.	The cost for training 200 staff nurses for 1 hour on the use of a congestive heart failure pathway resulted in 30 minutes of overtime for 60 staff members. 60 X 0.5 X $37.50= $1125.00.
One-time Benefits and Costs	One time benefits and costs need to be computed for the first year benefits and costs.	A construction project is canceled because of a reduction in the emergency department waiting time makes the construction un-necessary.

Terminology	Definition	Example
Centralized Costs	Consultants, training materials, facilities and equipment, supplies, and promotion or celebration costs.	An outside consultant on how to develop critical pathways.
Centralized Benefits	Income received from speaking and consulting fees and sale of materials developed.	After developing an automated nursing documentation system for homecare, the system was marketed to other agencies.

Once the decision rules are determined, it is time to estimate the financial costs and benefits of a quality or resource initiative. An example of a cost benefit analysis is shown below.

Cost Benefit Analysis of a Pneumonia Critical Pathway

♦ **Organizational Goals**
  - **Reduce the average length of stay from 6 days to 4 days.**
  - **Improve reimbursement**
  - **Reduce transfers to ICU**

♦ **Scope of Costs and Benefits (Marginal)**

Costs of Pathway	Benefits of Pathway
• Overtime for team meetings • Overtime for implementation training • Outside printing costs • Added staff for case management • Cost of food at meetings	• Reduction in the patient care costs • Increase in revenues • Sale of completed pathway

Pneumonia Benefit Analysis

- ◆ **Bacteria Pneumonia**
  - – 165 Cases a year
  - – Average cost of case: **$4000.00**
  - – Average reimbursement per case: ($500.00)
  - – Total profit/loss: ($82,500.00)
- ◆ **New Pathway**
  - – 165 Cases a year
  - – Average cost per case: $3300.00
  - – Average reimbursement per case: $200.00
  - – Total profit/loss: $33,000.00
- ◆ **Financial Benefits**
  - – Reduction or increase in cost: $ 700.00 per case
  - – $700 X 165 X 2 yrs = $231,000.00

Pneumonia Cost Analysis

- ◆ **Marginal Cost of Developing Pathway**
  - – Overtime for Staff: $0.00
  - – Overtime for Implementation Training: $500.00
  - – New Equipment: $0.00
  - – Printing Cost of Forms: $5000.00
  - – Food Costs: $300.00
- ◆ **Project Costs:** $5,800.00
- ◆ **Cost Benefit of Quality Initiative**
  - » $231,000.00 - $5,800.00 = $225,200

After the cost analysis is completed, a report highlighting all benefits, both tangible and intangible, needs to be written and submitted for review. The financial benefits and costs need to be reviewed by financial analysts and managers to obtain concurrence with the results.

Communicate, Communicate, Communicate

- ◆ Communicate widely so costs, benefits and returns are well understood
- ◆ Use multiple communication methods

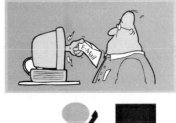

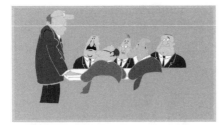

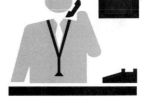

Cost-Benefit Analysis Worksheet

Cost of Old Process

1. Number of cases per year:_____

2. Average cost per case: $_____

3. Average reimbursement per case: $_____

4. Total profit / # of cases X (Avg. reimbursement - Avg. cost per case)

_____ X $_____ = $_____

Cost of New Process

1. Number of cases per year: _____

2. Average cost per case: $_____

3. Average reimbursement per case: $_____

4. Total profit / loss: # of cases X (Avg. reimbursement - Avg. cost per case)

_____ X $_____ = $_____

Financial Benefit:

1. Reduction or increase in cost: $_____

2. Difference in cost X # of cases X 2 yrs

   $_____ X _____ X 2 = $_____

Marginal Costs

1. Development Costs: $_____

2. Implementation Costs: $_____

3. Capital Cost Impact: $_____

4. Centralized Costs: $_____

5. Total Project Costs: $_____

Cost Benefit of Quality Initiative

1. Total Profit / Loss - Total Project Costs = Cost Benefit

   $_____ - $_____ = $_____

Appendix A
Exercise Answers

TABLE 7. Frequency Distribution Exercise: Page 14

Category	Frequency Distribution
Without Vasodilator	12
0-2 hours	3
Day 1	12
Day 2	3

TABLE 8. Arithmetic Mean Exercise: Page 17-18

Patient 2	2
Patient 3	7
Patient 6	7
Patient 9	5
Patient 13	9
Patient 15	8
Patient 18	5
Patient 23	6
Patient 26	5
Patient 27	7
Patient 29	9
TOTAL	70

$$\bar{x} = \frac{70}{11} = 6.36$$

TABLE 9. Geometric Mean Exercise: Page 18

Patients	LOS	logarithmic
Patient 2	2	
Patient 3	7	14
Patient 6	7	98
Patient 9	5	490
Patient 13	9	4410
Patient 15	8	35280
Patient 18	5	176400
Patient 23	6	1058400
Patient 26	5	5292000
Patient 27	7	37044000
Patient 29	9	333396000
TOTAL	70	

$GM = \sqrt[11]{3333960} = 5.9540788 = 5.95$

Median Exercise: Page 19

Step 1. 2,5,5,5,6,7,7,7,8,9,9

Step 2. 7

Step 3. 7

Range Exercise: Page 21

Step 1. 4,4,4,5,5,5,6,6,6,7,8,8,8,9,10,11

Step 2. 11-4=7

TABLE 10. Standard Deviation Exercise on Page 21-22

Patient	LOS	Avg. LOS	Deviation	Squared Deviation
1	5	6.08	-1.08	1.1664
4	4	6.08	-2.08	4.3264
7	6	6.08	-.08	0.0064
11	7	6.08	.92	0.8464
15	8	6.08	1.92	3.6864
16	4	6.08	-2.08	4.3264
19	3	6.08	-3.08	9.4864
20	11	6.08	4.92	24.2064
21	8	6.08	1.92	3.6864
24	5	6.08	-1.08	1.1664
25	6	6.08	-.08	0.0064
28	6	6.08	-.08	0.0064
TOTAL	73/ 12= 6.08			52.9168

Degree of freedom: 12-1 = 11

Variance: 52.9168/ 11 = 4.8106

$\sigma = \sqrt{4.8106} = 2.1933 = 2.19$

Z-score Exercise: Page 31.

Step 1. Mean =
2+7+8+7+5+7+10+9+5+4+6+5+3+8+5+5+7+4=107
/18 = 5.94

Step 2. SD = 2.10

Step 3. 6- 5.94 = 0.06

Step 4. z = 0.06 / 2.10 = 0.03

Chi square Exercise: Pages 33-36

Determine if there is a relationship between a patient being weighed (even one time) and having a length of stay of less than five days.

Step 1. Formulate a null and alternative hypothesis about the relationship between a treatment modality and the patient outcome.

Null: Weighing a CHF patient does not reduce the length of stay to below six days.

Alternative: Weighing a CHF patient reduces the length of stay to below six days.

Step 2. Select the desired level of significance 0.05

Step 3. Compute the degree of freedom for the test. (2-1) X (2-1) = 1

Step 4. Label each column with dependent outcomes and a column for total.

Step 5. Label each row with processes variables and a row for total.

Step 6. Place frequencies in the table for each event.

Step 7. Add all frequencies found in the rows and place in the total column.

Step 8. Add all frequencies found in the columns and place in the total row.

TABLE 15.

Step 4-8	LOS 5 Days or <	LOS of 6 Days or >	Total
Weighed	O = 8	O = 10	18
Not Weighed	O =5	O = 7	12
Total	13	17	30

This is observed frequency.

Step 9. Compute the expected probability for each cell by multiplying the row total by the column total and dividing by the grand total (Rule of Multiplication).

TABLE 12.

Step 9	LOS 5 Days or <	LOS 6 Days or >	Total
Weighed	$E = \left(\frac{13}{30} \times \frac{18}{30}\right) \times 30$ E = 7.8	$E = \left(\frac{17}{30} \times \frac{18}{30}\right) \times 30$ E = 10.2	18

TABLE 12.

Step 9	LOS 5 Days or <	LOS 6 Days or >	Total
Not Weighed	$E = \left(\frac{13}{30} \times \frac{12}{30}\right) \times 30$ E = 5.2	$E = \left(\frac{17}{30} \times \frac{12}{30}\right) \times 30$ E = 6.8	12
Total	13	17	30

Step 10. Subtract the expected frequency from the observed (O-E).

TABLE 13.

Step 10	LOS 5 Days or <	LOS 5 Days or >	Total
Weighed	8 - 7.8 = 0.2	10 - 10.2 = -0.2	18
Not Weighed	5 -5.2 = -0.2	7 - 6.8 = 0.2	12
Total	13	17	30

Step 11. Square the difference between the observed and the expected frequencies for each cell.

TABLE 14.

Step 11:	LOS 5 Days or <	LOS 6 Day or >	Total
Weighed	0.2^2 = 0.04	-0.2^2 = 0.04	18
Not Weighed	-0.2^2 = 0.04	0.2^2 = 0.04	12
	13	17	30

Step 12. Divide the squared value of each cell in step 11 by the expected value for the cell.

TABLE 15.

Step 12	LOS 5 Days or <	LOS 6 Days or >	Total
Weighed	0.04/ 7.8 =0.0051	0.04/ 10.2 =0.0039	18
Not Weighed	0.04/ 5.20.0076	0.04/ 6.80.0059	12
	13	17	30

Step 13.   0.0051 + 0.0039 + 0.0076 + 0.0059 = 0.0225

Step 14.   Critical Value = 3.841 > 0.0225

Conclusion: The null hypothesis cannot be rejected

Correlation Coefficient Exercise: Pages 44-47

Using the second case study, determine if there is a correlation between the number of chest x-rays and the length of stay.

Step 1.   Compute the mean for the first variable (x).

Step 2.   Compute the mean for the second variable (y).

Step 3.   Arrange the variables in corresponding rows in a table.

Step 4.   Subtract the answer from step 1 from each of the values in the first group of variables $(x - \bar{x})$.

Step 5.   Subtract the answer from step 2 from each of the values in the second group of variables $(y - \bar{y})$.

Step 6.   Multiply the results of step 4 by corresponding results from step 5.

TABLE 16.

Patient	X	Y	Step 4 $(x - \bar{x})$ (2.3)	Step 5 $(y - \bar{y})$ (5.6)	Step 6 $(x - \bar{x})(y - \bar{y})$	Step 8 $(x - \bar{x})^2$	Step 10 $(y - \bar{y})^2$
1	2	5	-0. 3	-0.6	0.18	0.09	0.36
2	3	7	0.7	1.4	0.98	0.49	1.96
3	1	4	-1.3	-1.6	2.08	1.69	2.56
4	1	6	-1.3	0.4	-0.52	1.69	0.16
5	2	5	-0.3	-0.6	0.18	0.09	0.36
6	4	9	1.7	3.4	5.78	2.89	11.56
7	4	7	1.7	1.4	2.38	2.89	1.96
8	2	4	-0.3	-1.6	0.48	0.09	2.56
9	2	5	-0.3	-0.6	0.18	0.09	0.36
10	3	6	0.7	0.4	0.28	0.49	0.16
11	4	6	1.7	0.4	0.68	2.89	0.16
12	1	5	-1.3	-0.6	0.78	1.69	0.36
13	2	4	-0.3	-1.6	0.48	0.09	2.56
14	3	4	0.7	-1.6	-1.12	0.49	2.56

TABLE 16.

Patient	X	Y	Step 4 $(x-\bar{x})$ (2.3)	Step 5 $(y-\bar{y})$ (5.6)	Step 6 $(x-\bar{x})(y-\bar{y})$	Step 8 $(x-\bar{x})^2$	Step 10 $(y-\bar{y})^2$
15	1	4	-1.3	-1.6	2.08	1.69	2.56
16	1	4	-1.3	-1.6	2.08	1.69	2.56
17	2	3	-0.3	-2.6	0.78	0.09	6.76
18	3	3	0.7	-2.6	-1.82	0.49	6.76
19	4	10	1.7	4.4	7.48	2.89	19.36
20	3	6	0.7	0.4	0.28	0.49	0.16
21	1	5	-1.3	-0.6	0.78	1.69	0.36
22	6	10	3.7	4.4	16.28	13.69	19.36
23	1	5	-1.3	-0.6	0.78	1.69	0.36
24	2	6	-0.3	0.4	-0.12	0.09	0.16
25	2	4	-0.3	-1.6	0.48	0.09	2.56
26	4	7	1.7	1.4	2.38	2.89	1.96
27	2	5	-0.3	-0.6	0.18	0.09	0.36
28	1	8	-1.3	2.4	-3.12	1.69	5.76
29	1	5	-1.3	-0.6	0.78	1.69	0.36
30	1	6	-1.3	0.4	-0.52	1.69	0.16
Total					Step 7: 41.6	Step 9: 48.3	Step 11: 97.2

Step 7. Add together all the products from step 6 .

Step 8. Square each difference computed in step 4.

Step 9. Add together each square computed in step 8.

Step 10. Square each difference computed in step 5.

Step 11. Add together each square computed in step 10.

Step 12. Compute the square root of the sum found in step 9.
$\sqrt{48.3} = 6.9498$

Step 13. Compute the square root of the sum found in step 11.
$\sqrt{97.2} = 9.859006$

Step 14. Multiply the square root found in step 12 by the square root found in step 13.

6.9498 X 9.859006 = 68.51812

Step 15. Divide the result from step 7 by the product of step 14.

41.6 / 68.51812 = 0.6071

Step 16. Determine the correlation between variables using Colton's rule of thumb shown below.

Correlation values	Degree of relationship
0 to 0.25 or 0 to -0.25	Little if any
.26 to 0.49 or -0.26 to -0.49	Low
0.50 to 0.69 or -0.50 to -0.69	Fair
0.70 to 0.89 or -0.70 to -0.89	High
0.90 to 1.00 or -0.90 to -1.00	Very High

Appendix B
Case Study Number 1

Hospital Anywhere has recently formulated a process improvement team to develop a systolic dysfunction congestive heart failure pathway. The pathway goals are the reduction of the average length of stay to four days and reduction of the pulmonary edema rate to three percent.

Based on these goals the team decided to collect data on the use of diuretics, vasodilators, diet therapy, and the assessment of patient weights. The results of this retrospective investigation are:

TABLE 17. Congestive Heart Failure Data

Patient	Diuretic	Vasodilator	Diet	Weighed	LOS	Pulm. Ed
1	Loop- 0-2hr	None	2 gm Na	None	5	None
2	Loop- 0-2hr	Isordil- Day 1	4 gm Na	Daily	2	None
3	Loop- Day 2	Nitro-0-2hr	4 gm Na	Day 2, 4,	7	Day 2
4	Loop- 0-2hr	None	Regular	None	4	None
5	Loop - Day 1	Isordil - Day 1	2 gm Na	Day 1	8	None
6	Loop- 0-2hr	Nitro/Isordil- Day 1	4 gm Na	Day 1, 3, 5	7	None
7	Loop- 0-2hr	None	Regular	None	6	None
8	None	None	Regular	Day 1	14	Day 4
9	Loop - Day 1	Nitro- Day 1	4 gm Na	Day 1	5	None
10	Loop- 0-2hr	None	2 gm Na	Day 1, 3	4	None

TABLE 17. Congestive Heart Failure Data

Patient	Diuretic	Vasodilator	Diet	Weighed	LOS	Pulm. Ed
11	Loop- Day 2	Nitro-0-2hr	Regular	None	7	Day 3
12	Loop - Day 1	Nitro/Isordil-Day 1	2 gm Na	Day 1, 2, 3, 4	10	None
13	Loop - Day 1	Nitro- Day 1	4 gm Na	Daily	9	None
14	Loop- 0-2hr	Nitro-0-2hr	Regular	Day 2	5	None
15	Loop - Day 1	None	4 gm Na	None	8	Day 4
16	Loop - Day 1	Nitro- Day 1	2 gm Na	None	4	None
17	Loop - Day 1	Isordil - Day 1	2 gm Na	Day 1	6	None
18	Loop - Day 1	Nitro/Isordil-Day 1	4 gm Na	Day 2	5	None
19	Loop- 0-2hr	Nitro- Day 1	2 gm Na	None	3	None
20	Loop - Day 1	None	Regular	None	11	None
21	Loop - Day 1	Nitro- Day 2	2 gm Na	None	8	None
22	Loop - Day 1	None	2 gm Na	Day 1	4	None
23	Loop - Day 1	None	4 gm Na	Day 2	6	None
24	Loop- 0-2hr	Nitro- Day 2	2 gm Na	None	5	None
25	Loop - Day 1	None	Regular	None	6	None
26	Loop - Day 1	Nitro- Day 2	4 gm Na	Daily	5	None
27	Loop - Day 1	Isordil - Day 1	4 gm Na	Day 1	7	None
28	Loop- 0-2hr	None	2 gm Na	None	6	None

TABLE 17. Congestive Heart Failure Data

Patient	Diuretic	Vasodilator	Diet	Weighed	LOS	Pulm. Ed
29	Loop - Day 1	Nitro- Day 1	4 gm Na	Daily	4	None
30	Loop- 0-2hr	None	Regular	Day 1	9	None

Case Study Number 2

The Medical Quality Improvement Committee at Hospital Anywhere has recently been investigating the treatment of Community Acquired Bacterial Pneumonia. The following data has been collected:

Patient	Antibiotic	Initial Timing (Elapsed time from Entry into ER)	Number of Chest X-rays	Co-Morbid Condition	LOS	Respiratory Failure
1	Rocephin	2 hr	2	CA Lung	5	No
2	Omnipen-N	6 hr	3	None	7	Day 2
3	Rocephin	1 hr	1	None	4	No
4	Omnipen	8 hr	1	None	6	No
5	Zinacef	2 hr	2	COPD	5	No
6	Recephin	10 hr	4	None	9	Day 2
7	Omnipen	4 hr	4	COPD	7	No
8	Unasyn	2 hr	2	None	4	No
9	Zinacef	12 hr	2	Alcohol dependent	5	Day 3
10	Principen	3 hr	3	None	6	No
11	Omnipen	5 hr	4	None	6	No
12	Rocephin	4 hr	1	Senile dementia	5	No
13	Rocephin	5 hr	2	None	4	No
14	Augmentin	2 hr	3	COPD	4	No
15	Omnipen	6 hr	1	None	4	No
16	Rocephin	3 hr	1	None	4	No
17	Zinacef	1 hr	2	None	3	No
18	Omnipen	0.5 hr	3	HPTN	3	No

Patient	Antibiotic	Initial Timing (Elapsed time from Entry into ER)	Number of Chest X-rays	Co-Morbid Condition	LO S	Respiratory Failure
19	Rocephin	8 hr	4	None	10	No
20	Rocephin	4 hr	3	HPTN	6	No
21	Piperacillin	3 hr	1	None	5	No
22	Rocephin	24 hr	6	CHF	10	Day 4
23	Rocephin	6 hr	1	None	5	No
24	Augmentin	8 hr	2	None	6	No
25	Bicillin	3 hr	2	CHF	4	No
26	Rocephin	4 hr	4	None	7	No
27	Unasyn	4 hr	2	COPD	5	No
28	Rocephin	5 hr	1	None	8	No
29	Unasyn	2 hr	1	None	5	No
30	Nafcillin	3 hr	1	COPD	6	No

Appendix C
Glossary of Terms

Alpha Error: Type I error. Rejecting a null hypothesis when it is true.

Alpha Value: The critical value level selected in a hypothesis test prior to performing the test.

Alternative Hypothesis: The opposite of the null hypothesis. It is the conclusion when the null hypothesis is rejected.

Analysis of Covariance: (ANCOVA) A special type of analysis of variance or regression used to control for the effect of a possible confounding factor.

Analysis of Variance: (ANOVA) A statistical procedure that determines whether or not there are any differences among two or more groups of subjects on one or more factors. The F test is used in ANOVA.

Bell-shaped distribution: A term used to describe the shape of the normal (Gaussian) distribution.

Beta Error: Type II Error. Not rejecting the null hypothesis when it is false.

Bias: The error related to the ways the targeted and sampled populations differ; it threatens the validity of a study. Bias can be either internal or external.

Categorical Observation: A variable whose values are classified into categories. Also known as nominal scale. This is generally considered qualitative data.

Central Limit Theorem: A theorem that states that the distribution of means is approximately normal if the sample size is large enough.

Chi-square Test: The statistical test used to test the null hypothesis that proportions are equal, that factors or characteristics are independent or not associated.

Cluster Random Sample: A two stage sampling process which first sub-divides the population into groups or clusters according to a specific characteristic, then a random sample of clusters is chosen. A portion of subjects within each cluster are selected. This sampling method is most often used in epidemiological research and commonly based on geographic areas or districts.

Coefficient of Determination: The square of the correlation coefficient. It is interpreted as the amount of variance in one variable that is accounted for by knowing the second variable.

Confidence Interval (CI): The interval computed from sample data that has a given probability that the unknown parameter, such as the mean or proportion, is contained within the interval. Common Confidence Intervals are 90 percent, 95 percent and 99 percent.

Confidence limits: The limits of a Confidence Interval. These limits are computed from sample data and have a given probability that the unknown parameter is located between them.

Contingency Table: A table used to display counts or frequencies for two or more nominal or quantitative variables.

Correlation Coefficient: A measure of the linear relationship between two numerical measurements made on the same set of subjects. It ranges from negative one (-1) to positive one (+1), with zero (0) indicating no relationship.

Critical Ratio: The term for the z-score used in statistical tests.

Critical Value: The value that a test statistic must exceed in order for the null hypothesis to be rejected.

Dependent Variable: An element in a study that's value is changed by the presence or absence of one or more other variables.

Distribution: The values of a characteristic or variable along with the frequency of their occurrence. Distributions may be based on empirical observations or may be theoretical probability distributions.

Dot Plot: A graphical method for displaying the frequency distribution of numerical observations for one or more groups.

Error Mean Square: The mean square in the denominator of F in ANOVA.

Event: A single outcome from an experiment.

Expected Frequencies: In contingency tables, the frequencies observed if the null hypothesis is true.

Factor: A characteristic that is the focus of inquiry in a study.

Factor Analysis: An advanced statistical method for analyzing the relationships among a set of items or indicators to determine the factors or dimensions that underlie them.

F Distribution: The probability distribution used to test the equality of two estimates of the variance. It is the distribution used with the F test in ANOVA.

Frequency: The number of times a given value of an observation occurs. It is also called counts.

Frequency Distribution: The list of values in a set of numerical observations that occur along with the frequency of their occurrence.

Geometric Mean: The nth root of the product of n observations. It is used with logarithms or skewed distributions.

Histogram: A graph of a frequency distribution of numerical observations.

Hypothesis: A statement describing a clinician's beliefs or educated guesses about the relationship between specific clinical elements and outcomes.

Hypothesis Test: An approach to statistical inference resulting in a decision to reject or not to reject the null hypothesis.

Independent Variable: A factor in a study that is unchanged by the presence or absence of other variables.

Intervention: The maneuver used in an experimental study. It may be drug or a procedure.

Kappa: A statistic used to measure interrater or intrarater agreement for nominal measures.

Level of Significance: The probability of incorrectly rejecting the null hypothesis in a test of hypothesis, also called alpha value or P-value.

Linear Regression: The process of determining a regression or prediction equation to predict Y from X.

Mean: The most common measure of central tendency. In a sample, the mean is the sum of the X values divided by the number in the sample.

Mean Square among Groups: An estimate of the variation in analysis of variance. It is the numerator of the F statistic.

Mean Square within Groups: An estimate of the variation in analysis of variance. It is the denominator of the F statistic.

Measures of Central Tendency: Summary numbers that describe the middle of a distribution.

Median: A measure of central tendency. It is the middle observation and is equal to the 50th percentile.

Mode: The value of a numerical variable that occurs the most frequently.

Multiple-comparison Procedure: A method for comparing several means.

Multiple Regression: A multivariate method for determining a regression or prediction equation to predict an outcome from a set of independent variables.

Multivariate: A term that refers to a study or analysis involving multiple independent or dependent variables.

Multivariate Analysis of Variance: (MANOVA) An advanced statistical method that provides a global test when there are multiple dependent variables and the independent variables are nominal.   It is analogous to analysis of variance with multiple outcome measures.

Nominal Scale: The simplest scale of measurement. It is used for characteristics that have no numerical values. It is also called a categorical or qualitative scale.

Nondirectional Test: A two-tailed test.

Null Hypothesis: The hypothesis being tested about a population. Null means no difference and refers to situations in which there is no difference.

Numerical Scale: The highest level of measurement. It is used for characteristics that can be given numerical values; the differences between numbers have meaning. Also called interval or ratio scale.

One-tailed Test: A test in which the alternative hypothesis specifies a deviation from the null hypothesis in one direction only. The critical region is located in one end of the distribution of the test statistic.

Ordinal Scale: Used for characteristics that have an underlying order to their values; the numbers used are arbitrary.

Parameter: The population value of a characteristic of a distribution.

Population: The entire collection of observation or subjects that have something in common and to which conclusions are inferred.

Power: The ability of a test statistic to detect a specified alternative hypothesis or difference of a specified size when the alternative hypothesis is true.

Probability: The number of times an outcome occurs in the total number of trials. If A is the outcome, the probability of A is denoted P(A).

P-value: The probability of observing a result as extreme as or more extreme than the one actually observed from chance alone.

Qualitative Observations: Characteristics measured on a nominal scale.

Quantitative Observations: Characteristics measured on a numerical scale; the resulting numbers have inherent meaning.

Range: The difference between the largest and the smallest observation.

Rank-order Scale: A scale for observations arranged according to their size, from lowest to highest or vice versa.

Simple Random Sample: A portion of items (cases) selected from a population in a manner which ensures all items have an equal chance or probability of being chosen.

Standard Deviation: The most common measure of dispersion or spread. It can be used with the mean to describe the distribution of observations.

Standard Error (SE): The standard deviation of the sampling distribution of a statistic.

Standard Error of the Mean: The standard deviation of the mean in a large number of samples.

Stratified Random Sample: Selecting a portion of a population by sub-dividing it according to specified characteristics, then randomly choosing cases from each sub-group.

Systematic Random Sample: A sampling method where every nth number of items is selected for the sample. "N" is a predetermined constant number of cases. For example, every seventh case will be included in the sample.

T Distribution: A symmetric distribution with mean zero (0) and a standard deviation larger than that for the normal distribution for small sample sizes.

T-test: The statistical test for comparing a mean with a norm or for comparing two means with small sample sizes. It is also used for testing whether a correlation coefficient or a regression coefficient is zero (0).

Two-tailed Test: A test in which the alternative hypothesis specifies a deviation from the null hypothesis in either direction. The critical region is located in both ends of the distribution of the test statistic.

Two-way Analysis of Variance: ANOVA with two independent variables.

Type I Error: The error that results if a true null hypothesis is rejected or if a difference is concluded when there is no difference.

Type II Error: The error that results if a false null hypothesis is not rejected or if a difference is not detected when there is a difference.

Variable: A characteristic of interest in a study that has different values for different subjects or objects.

Z-Approximation: The z-test is used to test the equality of two independent proportions.

Z-Ratio: The test statistic used in the z-test. It is formed by subtracting the hypothesized mean from the observed mean and dividing by the standard error of the mean.

Z-test: The statistical test for comparing a mean with a norm or comparing two means for large samples (n> 30).

Appendix D
Bibliography and
References

Association for Practitioners in Infection Control. *The APIC Curriculum for Infection Control Practice*. Dubuque: Kendall/Hunt, 1983. Vol. I.

Cook, Thomas D. and Campbell, Donald T. *Quasi-Experimentation: Design and Analysis Issues for Field Settings*. Boston: Houghton Mifflin Co, 1979.

Cryer, Jonathan D., and Miller, Robert B. *Statistics for Business: Data Analysis and Modeling*. Belmont: International Thomson Publishing, 1994.

Dawson-Saunders, Beth, and Trapp, Robert G. *Basic & Clinical Biostatistics*. Norwalk: Appleton & Lange, 1994.

Joseph, Eric D. *Statistical Imperative*. Chicago: Care Education Group, 1993.

Leedy, Paul D., *Practical Research Planning and Design*. New York: Macmillan , 1980.

Munro, Barbara Hazard and Page, Ellis Batten, *Statistical Methods: For Health Care Research*. 2nd Edition, Philadelphia: J.B. Lippincott, 1993.

Spiegel, Murray R. *Theory and Problems of Statistics*, 2nd Ed. New York: McGraw-hill, 1988.

Voelker, David H. and Orton, Peter Z. *Statistics*. Lincoln: Cliffs Notes, 1993.

Wall, Deborah K., and Proyect, Mitchell M. *Moving From Parameters To Pathways: A Guide For Developing And Implementing Critical Pathways*. Santa Cruz: Quality Team Associates, 1994.

Index